Keto After 50

The Ultimate Guide to Ketogenic Diet for Men and Women over 50 Including Cookbook with Mouthwatering Recipes to Accelerate Weight Loss and Reset Your Metabolism

Thomas Slow

TABLE OF CONTENTS

CHAPTER 3: OVERCOMING THE KETO FLU 75

CHAPTER 4: BASIC FITNESS FOR THE KETOGENIC DIET 90

CHAPTER 5: KETO RECIPES FOR BREAKFAST 99

CHAPTER 6: KETO RECIPES FOR LUNCH...............110

INTRODUCTION

Congratulations on purchasing *Keto After 50: The Ultimate Guide to Ketogenic Diet for Men and Women Over 50,* and thank you for doing so!

Before I started the Ketogenic Diet, I honestly struggled with my health and my lifestyle. I had no idea that the foods I was eating on a daily basis were slowly making me sicker by the day. While other diets had failed time and time again, I finally came across the Ketogenic Diet just before it was too late!

I decided to write this book to help people share the same success that I have. Through the science-backed Ketogenic Diet, I have lost thirty pounds and have changed my life for the better. While other diets have failed me, I have been following this lifestyle for five years now and will never go back!

That is one of the best parts of the Ketogenic Diet. While other diets are strict and hard to follow, the Ketogenic Diet is fairly basic once you grasp the basic concepts. Within the chapters of this book, you will find everything you need to know about the diet, including some tips and tricks I have learned along the way!

During my health journey, I hit just about every bump along the way. I have fallen off the ketosis-wagon time and time again. I hope that by preparing yourself with this book beforehand, you can get straight to the health benefits this diet has to offer! Honestly, it is one of the best decisions I have ever made for myself!

After you get through the basics of the diet and why it works for individuals, such as myself, over 50 years of age, you will be handed some of the most delicious recipes I have ever come across! Whether you are looking for a meal for lunch or dinner, I have got you covered! Yes, I have even included some of my favorite snacks and desserts for you to try because they are allowed and also encouraged on your new diet!

I hope that by the end of this book, you will feel like a Ketogenic Diet expert. As I said earlier, it changed my life for the better, and with some hard work and determination, it can change yours as well. When you are ready, we will start from the beginning of the diet.

CHAPTER 1: KETOGENIC DIET BASICS

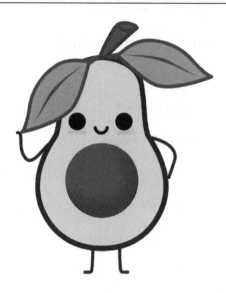

Before starting any diet, it is crucial you understand the history behind it. As you well know, there are many diets on the market in the modern age. The right question you need to ask for yourself is, Is the Ketogenic Diet right for you? Luckily for all of us, the Ketogenic Diet can help a wide range of individuals, whether you are young, older, or somewhere in between!

History of the Ketogenic Diet

The Ketogenic Diet first began in the 1920s and 30s. Initially, it was a popular therapy for individuals who had epilepsy. At the very beginning, the Ketogenic Diet was first developed to provide an alternative to fasting, which also worked well for epilepsy therapy.

While the diet did work for a while for these patients, it was eventually abandoned when modern medicine came around and was able to help a majority of patients with their symptoms. However, there were still approximately 30% of patients where the medication did not work, and the diet was re-introduced to help these individuals.

In 1921, it was an endocrinologist known as Rollin Woodyatt that was one of the first to notice the three water-soluble compounds that are produced in the liver when we are starved from carbohydrates. These three compounds are what we now know as ketone bodies. It was at this point, an individual from the Mayo Clinic known as Russel Wilder would call this "starvation from carbohydrates" as the Ketogenic Diet!

As the diet continues to grow in popularity, there is more research being performed on the Ketogenic Diet by the day!

With science-backed evidence, you can follow the diet and know for a fact that it is going to work.

How the Ketogenic Diet Works

Welcome to your first Ketogenic Diet Science lesson! One of the best parts of the Ketogenic Diet is the fact that it is based around a natural process that your body already has! The key to success is fueling your body correctly instead of stuffing it with overly-processed junk. In this guide, you will learn everything you need to know from what to eat when to eat and how to get into the best shape of your life!

The first lesson you need to know is that our body has four primary fuels that we use. These include glucose, protein, free fatty acids, and ketones. Each one of these fuel sources are stored in different proportions in our bodies. Overall, the fuel that we use the most is stored as triglyceride in our adipose tissue, aka, FAT! The second most used source is protein and glucose, which are used depending upon the metabolic state of your body.

So, what determines what fuel to use and when? As you might have already guessed, the primary determinant is based upon carbohydrate availability. Additional factors that can affect fuel utilization include a full or empty liver glycogen level and the levels of certain enzymes. Overall, total energy equals glucose plus FFA.

Next, it is vital that you understand that the body has three different fuel storages that it taps into when you begin to lower your calories. These three different storage depots include protein, carbohydrates, and fats! Protein is essential in your diet because it can be converted into glucose in your liver and then used as energy. Carbohydrates are typically stored as glycogen and are placed in your liver and muscle. Fat, on the other hand, is generally stored as body fat, but we will get to that in a second.

When you are following a SAD diet or a Standard American Diet, ketones truly have a non-existent role when it comes to your energy production. However, as you begin a ketogenic diet, it will play a much more significant role, and here we introduce the fourth potential fuel source for your body! As you start to decrease the carbohydrate availability through diet, your body will automatically make the shift to using fat as your first fuel source.

Health Benefits of the Ketogenic Diet

As you can tell, there are some extremely complex biological processes behind the Ketogenic Diet. When you first start this diet out, you will want to consult with a doctor before you begin any changes. As far as any diet goes, it is crucial that you choose one that is going to benefit you rather than do more harm. For this reason, be sure to consult with a professional before you experiment on yourself.

With that in mind, why begin any diet if it isn't going to benefit you? Before you dive into the diet itself, let's learn all of the incredible ways that the Ketogenic Diet can help you. Whether you are looking to lose weight, gain energy, or improve brain function, the ketogenic diet may be just what you were searching for.

Brain Benefits

As you begin to change the fuel source for your body, this includes significant fuel sources for your brain as well. Studies have found that through the Ketogenic Diet, individuals were able to increase the stability of their neurons as well as the up-regulation of the mitochondrial enzymes and brain mitochondria.

With that in mind, scientists have been studying how a Ketogenic Diet may be able to benefit those who have Alzheimer's disease. It seems as though through diet, individuals have been able to enhance their memory as well as increase cognition. When this happens, a diet may be able to bring improvement to individuals with all different stages of dementia.

For those who do not need to worry about Parkinson's disease or Alzheimer's Disease, the Ketogenic Diet is also <u>beneficial</u> in increasing mental focus, clarity, and could potentially grant less frequent and less intense migraines. Generally, these conditions are related to altered brain chemistry and stable blood sugar levels, both helped by the Ketogenic Diet.

Heart Disease

Another major benefit that makes people take a look at the Ketogenic Diet is the downstream effects of the diet on blood glucose levels. As you begin to cut carbohydrates from your diet, it can help keep your blood glucose stable and low. By doing this, individuals have been able to keep their blood pressure in check and are also able to lower their <u>triglyceride levels</u>.

When people first begin a Ketogenic Diet, they feel that it is counterintuitive to eat a higher percentage of fat in order to lower the triglycerides, but the truth is, fat has had a bad rep this whole time! In fact, it is eating excessive carbohydrates, especially fructose, that is the culprit behind increasing triglycerides! The truth is, through this new diet, you will be able to <u>raise</u> your good cholesterol and lower your bad cholesterol.

Fight Cancer

When it comes to cancer, it is essential that you seek medical attention before you try to take your life into your own hands through diet. It is highly advised that you listen to your doctor's advice when it comes down to cancer treatment. However, there have been articles published based around cancer and the ketogenic diet.

In 2014, Dom D'Agostino's lab published an <u>article</u> based around ketones being able to decrease tumor cell viability in mice that had metastatic cancer. Within this article, it was found that, generally, cancer cells will express an abnormal metabolism that is characterized when glucose consumption is increased. When this happens, the genes begin to mutate, and the mitochondrial begins to malfunction. In the studies, it is found that cancer cells are unable to use ketone bodies as energy, therefore inhibiting the viability of the tumor cell in the first place!

Improve Sleep and Energy Levels

Unfortunately, many individuals underestimate how important sleep is. The good news is that after only four or five days on the ketogenic diet, many individuals have reported that they already begin to benefit from higher energy levels. On a scientific level, this may be due to the fact that through your new ketogenic diet, you will be stabilizing your insulin levels. As your body becomes stabilized, this will help provide you with a ready source of energy rather than experiencing the spikes and crashes.

As far as sleeping goes, the ketogenic diet affects sleep are still being studied. Right now, it seems as though through diet, individuals are able to decrease the time they spend in REM and increase slow-wave sleep patterns. It is believed that this is due to a biochemical shift in the brain as your body learned to use ketones as energy. Either way, you will be sleeping more in-depth and longer than before, granting you a fresh start to each day!

Decrease Inflammation

Inflammation is a strange defense mechanism used in the body to help the immune system recognize any damaged cells, pathogens, or irritants. Through inflammation, the body is able to identify these issues and begin the healing process. While this is beneficial for the most part, it, unfortunately, can persist longer than needed and will end up causing more harm than good.

If you have inflammation in your body, you may experience symptoms such as pain, redness, swelling, immobility, and sometimes even heat. But, these signs of inflammations only apply to the inflammations on the skin. Sometimes, inflammation can happen within our internal organs, and that is when we experience symptoms such as fever, abdominal pain, chest pain, mouth sores, and even fatigue.

Studies have found that the key player in inflammation, and the diseases associated with it, is suppressed BHB. Luckily through the ketogenic diet, BHB is one of the primary ketones you will be producing as you begin your new diet. This meaning that you will be able to help issues, including IBS, eczema, psoriasis, acne, and even arthritis, all through diet!

Gastrointestinal and Gallbladder Health

If you suffer from heartburn or acid reflux on a daily basis, you may want to take a good, hard look at your diet. Unfortunately, many sugary foods, nightshade vegetables, and grain-based foods are major culprits of both heartburn and acid reflux. With that in mind, it shouldn't come as a surprise that when you change your diet to include low-carb foods, these symptoms will disappear almost instantly. The reason you experience these issues is through an autoimmune response, bacterial issue, and inflammation caused by these foods in the first place.

Another benefit of the Ketogenic Diet will be the altering of the microbiome found in your gut. An individual known as Dr. Eric Westman found that through diet, individuals are able to significantly reduce health issues as they change their microbiome. In fact, he believes that when you take away carbohydrates, this can fix just about any gastrointestinal issues that affect a number of different people.

Along those same lines, research has also found that carbohydrates may be a significant culprit behind gallstones as well. As far as the Ketogenic Diet goes, it appears that when individuals consume a diet that is higher in fat, this can help keep the system running smoothly and will prevent gallstones from forming in the first place.

Improved Kidney Function

Another common issue among the health community is kidney stones. The most common cause of both gout and kidney stones is due to elevated levels of phosphorus, oxalate, calcium, and uric acid in the body. Unfortunately, this is often combined with obesity, dehydration, bad genetics, sugar consumption, and alcohol consumption.

Through the Ketogenic diet, individuals are able to lower their uric acid levels and help improve the health of their kidneys. It should be noted that while the ketogenic diet can help long-term, this diet does temporarily raise the uric acid levels within the body, especially if you are dehydrated. While it does _rise_ as the ketone levels rise, the uric acid levels will lower in about four to six weeks.

Improved Women's Health

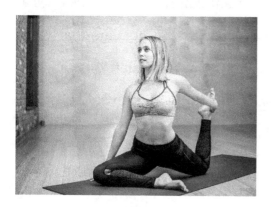

While the ketogenic diet is beneficial for both men and women, studies have shown that through diet, women may be able to stabilize their hormones and increase their fertility.

There was extensive <u>research</u> published in 2013 that looked at the key evidence linking ketogenic diets to enhancing fertility. It was also found that the Ketogenic Diet can treat PCOS (Polycystic Ovary Syndrome.) Through diet, individuals were able to eliminate or reduce <u>symptoms</u> of PCOS, including obesity, acne, and prolonged menstrual periods.

On a more general basis, it seems as though with this diet, individuals were able to keep their blood sugar levels low and stable. When this happens, it helps stabilize and equilibrate hormone levels, especially in women. Fortunately, this is a downstream benefit of the metabolic pathways that are related to insulin. Overall, individuals feel more balanced and stable than ever!

Improved Endurance and Muscle Gain

As we get older, we generally begin to lose the muscle mass we once had. As mentioned earlier, one of the main ketones you will begin producing as you begin the Ketogenic Diet is BHB. BHB is helpful in <u>promoting muscle gain</u>. When you combine the ketogenic diet with proper exercise, you will be increasing your health and muscle gain at the same time.

In addition to muscle gain, it is also believed that the diet can help improve endurance. Studies have found that athletes who switched to the diet and became fully fat-adapted showed significant improvements in both their mental and physical performances. Of course, this was compared to individuals who followed a typical diet that is rich in carbohydrates.

Weight Loss

Weight loss is one of the major reasons anyone begins a diet. Luckily through the ketogenic diet, there is substantial evidence that by eating the proper foods, you will be able to lose weight and preserve your muscle mass. In a related study, it was found that individuals who followed a ketogenic diet, compared to individuals on a low-calorie and low-fat diet were able to lose 2.2 times more weight! In addition, these people also improved their HDL cholesterol and Triglyceride levels.

The best part about losing weight on the Ketogenic diet is the fact that individuals are still able to lose fat without restricting their calories nor controlling their food intake. This is important to keep in mind when it comes down to sticking to any diet. When individuals hate the extra work of counting their calories, they are statistically more likely to return to their old eating habits. Later in this book, we will be going over the specifics of weight loss on the Ketogenic Diet.

Increased Metabolic Health

The last health benefit we will focus on in this chapter will be increased metabolic health. Metabolic syndrome is described as give common risk factors for heart disease, type 2 diabetes, and obesity. These include high blood sugar levels, low levels of HDL "good" cholesterol, high levels of LDL "bad" cholesterol, abdominal obesity, and high blood pressure. The good news is that many of these risk factors can be eliminated or improved through better lifestyle and nutritional changes.

An important factor behind these issues is insulin. Insulin plays a vital role as far as metabolic disease and diabetes go. Luckily, the Ketogenic Diet is very effective when it comes to lowering insulin levels for individuals who are prediabetic or have type 2 diabetes.

In one study, it was found that after only two weeks following the Ketogenic Diet, individuals were able to improve their insulin sensitivity by 75% and showed a blood sugar level drop from 7.5 mmol/l to a 6.2mmol/l! In another 16-week study, seven out of the 21 participants were able to stop their diabetic medication completely when they began the Ketogenic Diet.

As you can tell, the Ketogenic Diet can help a number of different people. While that is important to know, it is more important to understand how it works. The key to your success is going to be fat! While that may seem backward, what we are taught about fat is all backward! Yes, there are bad fats that we have to avoid, but good fat is going to be your new fuel source. Therefore, we will next learn the different types of fat you need to boost your success on the Ketogenic Diet.

Types of Fats for Ketosis

When you are following a Ketogenic Diet, about 70% of your calories will now be coming from fat sources. With that in mind, it can be hard figuring out which fats are healthy for you and which ones you should avoid. Below, you will learn the different types of fat you will be able to enjoy along with the keto-friendly sources you can find them in.

Good Fats

As a majority of fat is going to make up your new diet, it is important that you have a thorough understanding of the good fats that you will be able to enjoy.

The four main categories of fats that you will be picking from include saturated fats, polyunsaturated fats, monounsaturated fats, and naturally-occurring trans fats. Below, we will dive into each category to help give you a better idea of the fats you will want to keep an eye out for.

Saturated Fats

The most common misconception about fat circles around saturated fats. For years, this type of fat was believed to be harmful to the heart. In turn, the American Heart Association started the low-fat and fat-free craze in the 1970s. Luckily, recent studies have been debunking the claim that there is a link between disease and saturated fats. Instead, a balanced level of fat is now being linked to improved nutrition absorption, improved cognition, and balanced hormones.

One of the most popular types of saturated fat is medium-chain triglycerides. You probably know this more commonly as MCTs. MCTs can be found mainly in coconut oil but also is found in small amounts in palm oil and butter. The good news is that these saturated fats are easily digested by the body and get to the liver immediately for energy!

As you begin figuring out your diet, you will want to consider MCT oil. With this simple supplement, you can gain benefits such as boosting your immune system, suppressing your appetite, improving gut health, reducing the risk of heart disease, and even improving athletic performance. Saturated fat is also beneficial for enhancing your HDL and LDL cholesterol levels, maintaining bone density, and creating hormones such as testosterone and cortisol. Other good sources include:

- Cocoa Butter
- Heavy Cream
- Ghee
- Butter
- Red Meat
- Eggs

Monounsaturated Fats

The next type of fat we will be discussing are monounsaturated fats. Unlike with saturated fats, MUFAs have been known to be the healthy fat for a number of years now. MUFAs are linked to health benefits, such as increased insulin resistance and better cholesterol. This type of fat is also known to help lower blood pressure, lower an individual's risk for heart disease, and can even help reduce belly fat!

Luckily, MUFAs are found in a number of different healthy foods! Some of the more popular sources include:

- Avocados
- Avocado Oil
- Olive Oil
- Pecans
- Cashews
- Lard
- Bacon Fat

Polyunsaturated Fats

Here is when things can get a little tricky. When it comes to polyunsaturated fatty acids (PUFAs), it all comes down to how you use them. When polyunsaturated fats are heated, they form free radicals. Essentially, this means that this type of fat forms harmful compounds that can end up increasing your risk of cancer, cardiovascular disease, and inflammation. With that in mind, you will want to make sure that the sources of your PUFAs are cold and never used for cooking.

When appropriately used, PUFAs actually offer some great benefits. PUFAs provide you with essential nutrients of omega-3 and omega-6 fatty acids. Ideally, the radio of these should be around 1:1. On a standard western diet, the ratio of this is about 1:30. With that in mind, you will want to focus on PUFAs that are higher in omega-3s. Some of the benefits that come with proper levels of PUFAs include decreased risk of stroke, heart disease, autoimmune disorders, and inflammatory diseases. PUFAs also help reduce symptoms caused by depression and ADHD and improve overall mental health. Some of the healthy forms of PUFAs will be:

- Nut Butter
- Nuts
- Chia Seeds
- Sesame Oil
- Fish Oil
- Fatty Fish
- Sardines
- Flax Oil
- Walnuts
- Olive Oil

Natural Trans Fats

As far as good and bad fats go, trans fats can get a little tricky. A mass majority of trans fats are going to fall under the "bad" category, as they are harmful and unhealthy, but here we are discussing naturally occurring trans fats. This type of trans fat is known as vaccenic acid. Some of the health benefits that come along with vaccenic acid include reduced risk of heart disease, diabetes, and obesity. Naturally occurring trans fat could possibly protect against cancer as well. Generally, this type of trans fat is going to be found in grass-fed meats and dairy fats.

Bad Fats

As you can tell, there are many different types of dietary fats that you will be able to enjoy on the Ketogenic Diet. With all of the good in mind, now it is time to learn the types of fat you will want to either eliminate or reduce drastically in your new diet. Bad fats will slow down your weight loss process and could have adverse health effects. Luckily, there is power behind knowledge, and you will know the good and the bad before you even begin.

Polyunsaturated Fats and Processed Trans Fats

When people refer to "bad" fat, they are talking about processed trans fats. Unfortunately, this type of fat makes up a majority of consumed fats and are incredibly damaging to one's health. Generally, these artificial trans fats are formed during the production of food, through the processing of the polyunsaturated fats. For this reason, you will want to choose

PUFAs that have been unprocessed. As you will recall, heated PUFAs create harmful free radicals.

Some of the primary sources of trans fats come from hydrogenated oils that are found in fast food, crackers, cookies, margarine, and more. They are also found commonly in oils like canola, soybean, peanut, sunflower, and cottonseed. When this type of fat is consumed, it could increase your risk of certain cancers, heart disease, and your LDL levels. Trans fats also increase body fat and lead to unwanted weight gain. Overall, you will want to learn how to reduce this fat in your diet so you can benefit from the good fats.

Plant-based Fats

Later in this book, you will learn that there are several different types of the Ketogenic Diet. Some individuals choose to follow a Vegan Ketogenic Diet. Therefore, I feel it was important to include a section based around plant-based fats. It does become slightly more complicated, but there are definitely sources of fat out there that are plant-based.

1. Nuts

    The diet industry has gone back and forth whether nuts are healthy for us or not. Luckily, on the Ketogenic Diet, nuts are an excellent source of both protein and monounsaturated fats. Some of the better nuts for you to incorporate into your diet will be Brazil nuts, almonds, and walnuts.

2. Seeds

Another common source of protein for you to consider will be seeds! Seeds are great because they can be sprinkled on anything from breads to sweets to salads! Seeds such as hemp seeds and chia seeds have an excellent source of omega-3 fatty acids, and sunflower seeds provide monounsaturated fats.

3. Avocados

Avocados have been growing in popularity by the day! Avocados are packed with monounsaturated fats and can be very versatile when it comes to cooking. Whether you enjoy guacamole or chocolate mousse, there are many different ways to pack extra good fats into your diet.

4. Coconut Oil

One of the more common ways to incorporate plant-based fats into your diet will be through coconut oil. Coconut oil offers delicious flavors, can handle high temperatures, and offers those MCTs we discussed earlier.

5. Cacao Nibs

Yes, chocolate is now considered a health food! However, it is important to avoid the chocolate that is found in candy bars; that type of chocolate is full of sugar and bad for your health. It turns out that dark chocolate offers both monounsaturated fats and anti-oxidants! While, of course, it is essential to keep any fat in moderation, it is good to have on hand!

Quick Start Guide for the Ketogenic Diet

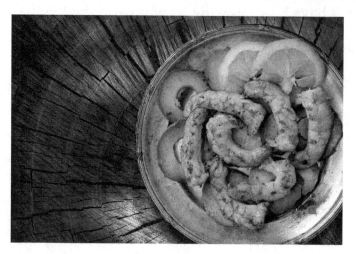

For those of you who are anxious to get started, there are a few basic rules you will want to follow when it comes to the Ketogenic Diet.

Good-bye Carbs

The golden rule to follow when starting your diet will be cutting the carbs! Later in the book, we will be going over macronutrients and how this pertains to your diet. For now, you will want to aim for your carb count to be 30 grams or under.

Eat Your Vegetables

As you learn to incorporate more fats into your diet, it should be kept in mind that fats are going to be higher in calories. If you are looking for weight loss on the Ketogenic Diet, you will want to make sure you are eating plenty of low-carb veggies to lower your overall caloric intake for the day. By doing this, you will be able to fill your plate and your stomach.

Make a Plan

When you first begin any diet, it can be hard to know where to start. Before starting the Ketogenic Diet, you will want to do some research to help you find low-carb meals for the week. Luckily within the chapters of this book, you will be provided with both recipes and a plan!

Trial and Error

On the Ketogenic Diet, there is going to be plenty of trial and error. The experimenting is half of the fun! While you will need to cut down on the carbs, there are plenty of other foods that you will be able to enjoy and are encouraged to try them all! Eventually, you will find your staples, and you will become a Ketogenic Pro!

Track Your Progress

This is honestly one of my favorite parts of starting the Ketogenic Diet. You may be reluctant to do this at first, but I promise that as the results begin rolling in, you will want to see how far you have come! Whether you take measurements, photos, or simply monitor your weight, you will want to continue doing this every three to four weeks. After a month alone, you may be pleasantly surprised just how far you have come.

Of course, there is much more to the Ketogenic Diet than this quick list, but it is an excellent place to get started. To further your knowledge on the subject, be sure to read the rest of this book!

Common Mistakes to Avoid

As you are well aware of at this point, there are some incredible benefits that come with the Ketogenic Diet. When you first start this diet, you are going to make a number of different mistakes. Whether you eat too many carbs, fall out of ketosis, or even just ditch your entire diet for the day, that is okay! What isn't okay is giving up this diet for good. Luckily because you are here, you will now learn some of the common mistakes people make on the Ketogenic Diet and how to avoid them in the first place!

Excess Protein

Excess protein intake is probably one of the biggest mistakes individuals make on this diet, especially when they are first getting started on the Ketogenic Diet. This is due to the fact that individuals give too much credit to the process of gluconeogenesis. You may be asking yourself, gluco-what? The method of gluconeogenesis is the process where your liver converts the protein you consume into blood glucose.

The key here is to realize that gluconeogenesis will only operate when it is on-demand, not when it is available. Essentially, this means that just because you ate a lot of protein in one day does not mean that it will automatically be converted into glucose. This process will only occur if your body needs glucose in the first place. So, while protein is going to be necessary on your diet, it should be consumed in moderation.

Excess Nuts and Dairy

As you learned earlier, dairy and nuts are both going to be significant sources of fats, but with that in mind, remember that these two foods are both calorie-dense. For this reason, it can become incredibly easy to overindulge on these foods, causing weight gain. Much like with protein, you can still enjoy these foods, but in moderation. If you feel dairy and nuts are trigger foods for you, you may want to try avoiding them for the first few weeks that you are following a Ketogenic Diet.

Adaption Time

While starting any diet, it is important not to expect results overnight. As you begin the Ketogenic Diet, you are going to be putting your body through some pretty profound changes. With such a significant difference, may come considerable struggles. Luckily, our bodies are pretty hardy when it comes to dealing with change and adapting to a different diet. It may seem frustrating at first, but you need to give your body time to adjust to your new diet. Remember that you are not just changing your diet; you are changing your overall fuel source!

Give yourself some time, and the benefits will come before you know it.

Excess Carbohydrates

At this point, you are well aware that the Ketogenic Diet is based around limiting carbs. Unfortunately, this can be very tricky when you are first starting out. As you learn what you can and cannot eat, you can expect to be in and out of ketosis fairly often. While this may be frustrating, you may want to take a closer look at your diet.

The key here is figuring out the maximum net carbs you can have in a day, depending on your activity level and metabolism. In the chapter to follow, we will be going more into depth on this subject. For general purposes, you will want to stay below 20 net carbs in a day to help you stay in ketosis. Once you become adapted to your new diet, you will learn precisely what your personal limit is and will excel from that point.

Snacking

In general, it is a pretty common habit to snack throughout the day. For some, this is to cure anxiety, and for others, its due to pure boredom! Snacking is also included in a number of different leisure activities, from dining out with friends to simply watching a movie.

If you are looking to lose weight on the Ketogenic Diet, you may want to limit your snacking. No matter what diet you follow, weight loss is equal to burning more calories than you consume. This rule is no different on your new diet.

Dehydration and Electrolytes

In the third chapter of this book, we will be tackling the dreaded Keto Flu. When you are first starting out, you will want to make sure you are staying hydrated and getting in enough electrolytes. The ketogenic diet has a dietetic effect, and when you lose water, you lose electrolytes. The three electrolytes you will want to focus on include magnesium, potassium, and sodium. Some of the best sources of potassium will be salmon, broccoli, spinach, and avocado. As long as you keep water and electrolytes consumption up, it will help you drastically while dealing with the symptoms of the Keto Flu.

Mindset

Finally, the most prominent mistake people make it not having the right mindset. If you are negative and miserable about your new diet, there is no way that you are going to stick with it! Instead, try your best to have a winner's mindset. This meaning that you start the diet off with clear goals and a reason behind your why. As you begin, ask yourself what is motivating you to begin this diet in the first place. What is going to drive you? Who are you doing this for? When you want to succeed at this diet more than anything else in the world, that is where you will find your success.

Now that you have a thorough understanding of Ketogenic Basics, it is time to learn how the Ketogenic Diet can help those of us who are over the age of 50! Yes, we are getting older, but life isn't over yet! There are still plenty of reasons to boost our health and perhaps live even better than when we were younger. If that sounds good to you, let's dive right into the next chapter.

CHAPTER 2: KETOGENIC DIET AFTER 50

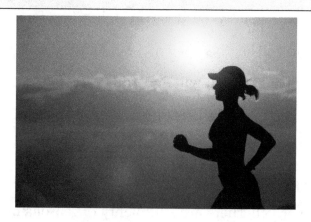

At any age, proper nutrition is incredibly important, but as we age, our bodies are going through some major changes. To help with these changes, it will be essential to make certain adjustments to our routines and nutrition. The vital factor to remember is that it is never too late to start taking care of yourself. When you neglect your health after the age of fifty, the effects may become more noticeable than ever before. So, how exactly does age affect our nutritional needs?

Aging and Nutritional Needs

As we age, you can expect a number of different changes to happen in your body, including thinner skin, loss of muscle, and less stomach acid. When these things happen, this can, unfortunately, make you more prone to nutrient deficiencies and overall quality of life. This is where the Ketogenic Diet comes in handy! By eating a variety of foods and incorporating the proper supplements, you will be able to meet your nutrient needs with no issues! Below, you will find some of the effects of aging and how to help the issue.

Less Calories- More Nutrients

On a general basis, an individual's daily calorie count will depend on a number of factors, including activity level, muscle mass, weight, and height. As for us older adults, we will need to begin lowering the number of calories we take in, in order to maintain or lose weight. Generally, older adults tend to exercise and move less compared to younger individuals.

While consuming fewer calories, it is important to continue getting higher levels of nutrients. For this reason, it is highly suggested to consume a variety of foods such as low-carb vegetables and lean meats to help get the proper nutrients and fight against any nutrient deficiencies. The nutrients you will want to focus on include vitamin B12, calcium, and vitamin D, Magnesium, Potassium, Omega-3 fatty acids, and Iron.

Benefits of Fiber

While many people do not like to discuss this, constipation is a prevalent health issue for individuals over the age of 50. In fact, women over the age of 65 are two to three times more likely to experience constipation! This may be due to the fact that people over the age of 50 generally move less and are more likely to be taking a medication that has constipation as an unfortunate side effect.

To help relieve constipation, you will want to make sure you are getting enough fiber. When you eat more fiber, it is able to pass through your gut, undigested, and help regulate bowel movements and form stool. As an added benefit, high-fiber diets may also be able to prevent diverticular disease. Diverticular disease is a condition where small pouches build along the wall of the colon and become inflamed.

Focus on Protein

In the chapter above, you learned that it is important not to focus on protein, but it will be essential to find a balance on your new diet. As we age, it is very common to lose both strength and muscle. In fact, on average, an adult will lose anywhere between 3-8% of their muscle mass per decade after the age of 30. When we lose muscle mass, it could lead to poor health, fractures, and weakness among an elderly population.

By eating more protein, you can help fight sarcopenia and maintain your muscle mass.

Vitamin B12

As mentioned earlier, keeping up with proper nutrients is going to be vital for your health. One of the vitamins you will want to focus on is Vitamin B12. This is a water-soluble vitamin that is in charge of making red blood cells and keeping your brain healthy. Unfortunately, it is estimated that anywhere from 1—30% of individuals over the age of 50 have a lowered ability to absorb this vitamin from their diet.

One of the main reasons individuals over the age of 50 have difficulty absorbing vitamin B12 may be due to the fact that they have reduced stomach acid reduction. Vitamin B12 is bound to proteins. In order for your body to use this vitamin, the stomach acid separates it from the protein and becomes absorbed. To benefit your new diet, you will want to consider taking a supplement of vitamin B12 or consuming foods that are fortified with the vitamin.

Vitamin D and Calcium

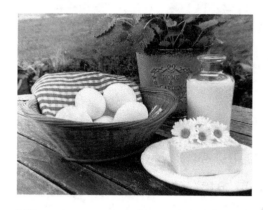

When it comes to bone health, calcium and vitamin D are going to be very important. While calcium is in charge of maintaining and building healthy bones, it depends on vitamin D to help the body absorb the calcium in the first place! Unfortunately, adults have a harder time absorbing calcium in their diets. This may be due to the fact that the gut absorbs less calcium as we age. However, the main culprit of a reduction in calcium is typically due to a vitamin D deficiency. As you can tell, they work hand in hand!

The reason we may experience a vitamin D deficiency is due to thinning skin. Generally, our body makes vitamin D from the cholesterol in the skin when it is exposed to sunlight. As the skin becomes thinner, it reduces the ability to make vitamin D and, in turn, reduces the ability to get enough calcium. When these two things happen, it increases the risk of fractures and bone loss.

To help counter this aging effect, you will want to make sure you are getting enough vitamin D and calcium in your diet. Some accessible sources will be dairy products, leafy vegetables, and dark greens. As far as Vitamin D goes, you will want to include a variety of fish or even a Vitamin D supplement such as cod liver oil.

Dehydration

On the Ketogenic Diet or not, staying hydrated is important at any age. In fact, water makes up about 60% of our bodies! Whether you are 20,30, or 50, the body still continually loses water through urine and sweat. As we age, it makes us more prone to dehydration.

When we become dehydrated, the water detects the thirst through receptors found all throughout the body and the brain. As we age, the receptors become less sensitive, making it hard to distinguish the thirst in the first place. On top of this, our kidneys are there to help converse water, but they also lose function with age.

Unfortunately, the consequences of dehydration are pretty harsh for the older population. When you are dehydrated long-term, this could reduce your ability to absorb medication and could worsen any medical condition. For this reason, it will be vital you keep up with your intake of water. I suggest trying a water challenge with friends and family or try having a glass of water with each meal you have.

Appetite

One of the last topics we will tackle on the subject of aging it the decrease in appetite. While this may seem like a benefit, a lack of eating could lead to a number of different nutritional deficiencies and unwanted weight loss. Poor appetite is most commonly linked to a heightened risk of death and overall poor health.

It is believed that some of the significant factors behind appetite loss could be due to changes in smell, taste, and hormones. Generally, older adults who have lower levels of hunger have higher levels of fullness hormones. When this happens, it causes individuals to be less hungry overall. As we age, the changes in smell and taste can also make food seem less appealing.

If you find this happens to you, you may want to establish a healthy habit of snacking. When you snack, try to reach for keto-friendly foods such as eggs, yogurt, and almonds to help put the nutrients back into your diet. If you are aware of this issue, it is something you can get a grasp on before it becomes a real problem.

Ketogenic Diet Changes for Aging Adults

As far as aging and nutrition go, it all comes down to a proper diet to help fuel you. The good news is that keto-friendly foods generally offer higher nutrition per calorie. This is vital as you already know that your basal metabolic rate is going to drop as you get older. Remember, the key here is to take in fewer calories but the same or more amount of nutrients! When you eat foods that are fighting disease and supporting your health, this will help you enjoy your golden years to the fullest.

The central concept you will want to promote for your new diet is to avoid empty calories. Empty calories generally come from foods that are high in sugars or lack nutrients, to begin with. You may have been able to live off junk food in your 20s, but you can kiss those days goodbye. Now, it is time to fill your plate with nutrient-dense foods.

No matter what your age is, it is never a bad idea to improve your health through diet. It is never too late to begin, and the sooner you start, the sooner you will feel better! The Ketogenic diet is meant for longevity. At this prime age, you will want to stop with the fad diets. They may work for a while, but it isn't worth doing if you aren't going to stick with the diet. Through the Ketogenic diet, you will be able to support your immunity, blood sugar levels, and put yourself at a healthier weight. If that all sounds good to you, let's take a look at what you can and cannot eat while following the Ketogenic Diet.

Foods to Enjoy

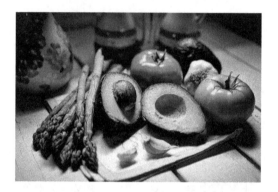

While starting a new diet can seem challenging enough, it is even harder when you are not sure what you can and cannot eat. Luckily, you will now find a comprehensive list of foods you will be able to enjoy while following a Ketogenic Diet. As you will soon find out, there is a wide variety of foods you will be able o enjoy, even if you are losing your beloved carbs.

Fats and Oils

As you already know, fats are now going to make up a majority of your calories in a day. The good news is that there a number of different ways to incorporate fats into your diet, whether you want to consume them as a dressing, sauce, or part of any meal!

When you are choosing fats for your diet, remember that eating the wrong type of fat can be dangerous for your health. As a quick recap, you will want to eat foods that have saturated, monounsaturated, and polyunsaturated fats while avoiding processed trans fats. This can be easily accomplished whether you are cooking with coconut oil, lard, or even tallow. Another factor on the Ketogenic Diet to keep in mind will be balancing your omega 3 fatty acids and your omega 6 fatty acids. As you will recall from earlier, these are found in food sources such as shellfish, trout, tuna, and even salmon. These essential fatty acids are necessary for your health, but it is important to find that balance. Below, you will find a thorough list of foods that will provide the best sources of fats for your diet.

- MCT Oil
- Macadamia Oil
- Avocado Oil
- Coconut Oil
- Coconut Butter
- Ghee

- Butter

- Brazil Nuts

- Avocados

- Lard

- Fatty Fish

- Non-hydrogenated Animal Fat

- Egg Yolks

- Tallow

- Mayonnaise

- Cocoa Butter

- Olive Oil

Protein

When it comes to protein on the Ketogenic Diet, you will want to try your best to keep your portions in moderation. As you shop around for your protein sources, your best bet will be choosing protein that has been grass-fed and pasture-raised. By doing this, you will be able to minimize the intake of steroid hormones and bacteria.

As far as red meat goes, you pretty much can't go wrong! There are some cured meats and sausages that have added ingredients, but it is easy enough to avoid these. Instead, stick with fattier cuts of steak such a ribeye or fatty ratios of ground beef. Just remember that when you are incorporating protein into your diet, too much protein could kick you out of ketosis.

In order to balance the protein in your meals, you can pair them with a fatty sauce or side dish. Some of the best sources of proteins include:

- Nut Butters
- When you shop for nut butter, be sure that they are unsweetened and natural. Generally, you will want to stick with macadamia or almond butter instead of peanut butter.
- Pork

  There are many different types of pork for you to enjoy from ham, tenderloin, pork chops, pork loin, or even ground pork. When picking out pork, be sure to avoid added sugars and get the fattiest cuts possible.
- Beef

  Beef is excellent to include on the Ketogenic Diet because it is incredibly versatile. When picking out beef, try to get fattier cuts of stew meat, roasts, steak, and ground beef.
- Eggs

Another excellent source of protein is going to come from whole eggs. These are great to have on hand because you can enjoy them in a number of different ways, from scrambled, poached, boiled, or even fried. When shopping for eggs, try to find them free-range.

- Shellfish & Fish

Finally, seafood is going to be an excellent source of protein for you. When shopping for fish, you will want to lean toward a selection that has been wild-caught. Look for fattier fish such as tuna, trout, snapper, salmon, mackerel, flounder, cod, and even catfish. As far as seafood goes, you can enjoy squid, mussels, scallops, crab, lobster, and even clams!

Fruits and Vegetables

Up until this point, you have probably learned that a balanced diet incorporates plenty of fruits and vegetables. While these are important for a balanced diet, some vegetables are high in sugar and low in nutrition. On the Ketogenic Diet, you will be consuming vegetables that are low in carbohydrates but still high in nutrients.

To stay on the safe side of vegetable selection, the secret to shopping will be sticking with vegetables that are grown above ground. Generally, these vegetables will be green, dark, and leafy. As you shop for your vegetables, you will want to opt for organic when possible, to help avoid pesticide residue. If you do find a vegetable that is grown below ground, this can still be enjoyed but in moderation. Below, you will find some low-carb vegetables for you to try.

- Spinach
- Baby Bella Mushrooms
- Green Bell Peppers
- Green Beans
- Romaine Lettuce
- Cabbage
- Cauliflower
- Broccoli
- Yellow Onion

As far as fruits go, these will generally be nonexistent on the Ketogenic Diet. Unfortunately, fruits typically have a higher carb count and are high in natural sugars. If you still crave some fruit, you can enjoy a limited amount of berries such as blueberries, blackberries, and raspberries. For cooking, you can also enjoy a limited amount of fresh lime and lemon juice.

Nuts and Seeds

Nuts are great to have on hand because they are an excellent source of fats, but remember to keep these in moderation because the carb count can add up quickly. You may also want to consider roasting the seeds and nuts to remove any anti-nutrients before enjoying it. Either way, raw nuts are great when you are looking to add texture or flavor to any meal. Nuts are also great for a quick snack.

As you choose your nuts, you will want to select from the following:

- Low Carb Nuts
- Some fatty, low carb nuts you will want to consider for your diet will be pecans, brazil nuts, and macadamia nuts. These are great to add a supplement of fat to your diet
- Moderate Carb Nuts

  Next, we have the fatty, moderate carb nuts. These include pine nuts, peanuts, hazelnuts, almonds, and walnuts. These can be added for flavor and texture but should be enjoyed in moderation.
- High Carb Nuts

The nuts you will want to avoid on the Ketogenic Diet will be cashews and pistachios. These are very high in carbohydrates and can easily kick you out of ketosis.

Dairy Products

As you begin the Ketogenic Diet, you will want a majority of your meals to come from fats, vegetables, and proteins. With that in mind, it is perfectly okay to enjoy dairy products in moderation. In general, you will want to make sure these products are organic or even raw. Unfortunately, dairy products that have been highly processed can contain anywhere from two to three times the amount of carbohydrates compared to the organic version. With that in mind, you will also want to choose products that are full fat. Some popular products include:

- Mayonnaise
- Hard Cheese
- Soft Cheese
- Whipping Cream
- Greek Yogurt

If you are looking to lose weight on the diet, it should be noted that some people have experienced slower weight loss when they ate too many dairy products. While it is okay to enjoy your share of cheese, you will want to keep dairy products in moderation. If you notice a slow down or plateau in your weight loss journey, cutting dairy would be a smart move to see if that is the culprit.

Cooking Flours

As you will find in a number of different recipes, cooking flours are going to be important to have on hand. Luckily, there are plenty of seed and nut flours for you to try out instead of regular flour. With that in mind, it will still be vital that you eat these in moderation.

Once you have become more comfortable with the Ketogenic Diet, you will learn how to combine multiple flours to get a better texture while baking. As you combine flowers, this can help you lower your net carbs if you are baking your own foods. You will want to keep in mind that these different flours do act in different ways. As an example, if you are cooking with coconut flour, you will want to use half the amount you would if you were using almond flour. Some of the more popular baking flours include:

- Flaxseed Meal
- Chia Seed Meal
- Coconut Flour

- Almond Flour

- Unsweetened Coconut

Spices and Condiments

Surprisingly enough, sauces and seasonings can be a very tricky part of the Ketogenic Diet. While many individuals freely use spices to add flavor to their meals, this is a sure way to add carbohydrates and processed ingredients without even knowing it!

While spices do have carbs in them, you will want to make sure you are counting them along the way. With that in mind, it should be noted that most of the pre-made spice mixes have added sugar. For this reason, you will want to make sure that you read any nutrition labels before you use or purchase an item. Below, you will find a list of common spices people still incorporate on their Ketogenic Diet.

- Pepper

- Sea Salt

- Thyme

- Rosemary

- Parsley

- Cilantro

- Oregano

- Cumin

- Basil

- Cinnamon

- Cayenne Pepper

- Chili Powder

When it comes to condiments and sauces, there seems to be a gray area on the Ketogenic Diet. If you want to be strict, you will want to avoid condiments and sauces as much as you can. Unfortunately, many of the pre-made condiments and sauces have added sweeteners or sugars that aren't keto-friendly. However, you can still make your own versions and avoid the excess carbs and sugars.

If you are desperate you can use some of the following in moderation:

- Ranch Dressing

- Yellow Mustard

- Low-sugar Ketchup

- Sriracha

- Vinaigrette Dressing

- Mayonnaise

- Soy Sauce

- Hot Sauce

- Horseradish

- Relish

- Sauerkraut

Sweeteners

When you first begin the Ketogenic Diet, it may be a good idea to stay away from sweet foods. By doing this, it can help keep your cravings to a minimum and can boost your success on the diet. However, if you genuinely need something sweet, it is better to have keto-friendly options to choose from.

As you begin searching for keto-friendly sweeteners, you will want to try to find one that is a liquid version. By doing this, you can avoid binders such as maltodextrin and dextrose that are higher in carbohydrates. Luckily, there are several sweeteners on the market that have a low glycemic impact. Some of the more popular sweeteners include:

- Stevia

- Monk Fruit

- Sucralose

- Erythritol

Beverages

Last but not least, we have keto-friendly beverages! As you learned earlier, the ketogenic diet has a natural diuretic effect. If you are just starting the diet, dehydration is a very common symptom to experience. On average, you will want to try your best to drink upward toward a gallon of water per day.

While water is important, it can become quite dull if it is the only liquid you are drinking. Another popular beverage people enjoy on the Ketogenic Diet is tea or Ketoproof coffee. Ketoproof coffee is excellent to have on hand to give you a boost of fat in the morning. Some other popular beverage choices include:

- Water, Water, and More Water!
- Broth
- Coffee
- Tea
- Almond Milk
- Coconut Milk

Foods to Avoid

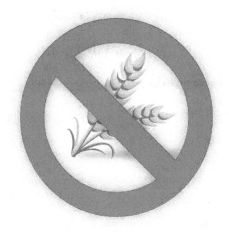

With a thorough understanding of the foods that you get to enjoy on the Ketogenic diet, it will be pretty easy to understand the foods that you will want to eliminate or avoid. If you are still unsure about any food items, it is probably safe to assume that they are not keto-friendly. While we want to focus on the positives of the Keto-genic diet, below you will find a list of foods you should avoid when you can.

Grains

This should be pretty much a given as you begin the Ketogenic Diet. Any wheat products such as beer, corn, rice, cakes, cereal, pasta, or bread need to be avoided on the Keto diet. It does not matter if it is made from quinoa, buckwheat, barley, rye, or wheat; these products are all going to be way too high in carbs.

Sugar

Much like with carbohydrates, you will want to avoid foods that are high in sugar. Typically, this means anything from ice cream, chocolate, candy, juice, soda, and even sports drinks. If it is processed and sweet, throw it out!

Low-fat Foods

As a society, we have been brainwashed to believe that low-fat foods are good for us! Unfortunately, these foods often have higher sugar and carb counts compared to the full-fat version. If you see low-fat on a package, it is best to leave it at the store.

Starch

While some vegetables are going to be tempting, it is best to stick with the list of approved vegetables in the section above. Some vegetables, such as potatoes and yams, are going to be too high in carbohydrates for the Ketogenic Diet. You will also want to avoid products like muesli and oats as well.

Fruits

Finally, you will want to avoid large fruits as well as you begin your diet. Anything from apples to bananas and oranges is going to be high in sugar and unnecessary for your diet. As mentioned earlier, you will still be able to consume berries in moderation.

As you can tell, there are plenty of foods that you will be able to enjoy on the Ketogenic Diet. While it will take quite a bit of trial and error, you will eventually find the foods that you truly enjoy, and you can make them staples in your daily diet.

Next on our list, it is time to learn about macronutrients. This is a vital lesson for anyone because your goals will be based on your macros, especially when you are trying to find your sweet spot for carbohydrates. When you are ready, let's move onto our next lesson.

Macronutrients 101

Whether you are looking to gain, lose, or maintain your weight, it will be important to understand what macronutrients are when starting a Ketogenic Diet. As you may already know, you will need to consume fewer calories when you are trying to lose weight and eat more if you are looking to gain weight. While it will take some time to figure out what your body needs, you will eventually find the sweet spot to achieve optimal health.

Macronutrients

You have probably heard of macronutrients before, but what are they exactly? Macronutrients are an organic or chemical compound that are consumed to give us the nutritional value and energy we need in order to survive. The macronutrients include proteins, carbohydrates, and fats.

- 1g of Carbs= 4 Calories
- 1g of Fat=9 Calories
- 1g of Protein=4 Calories

Fats

The first macronutrient we will discuss is fats. As you already know, there are unsaturated and saturated fats. This nutrient is essential because Vitamins K, E,D, and A can only be consumed in this form. On the Ketogenic Diet, around 70% of your calories will be coming from fat.

Protein

Next, we have Protein. Protein can be composed of several different types of amino acids and are the "building blocks" of the human body. Interestingly enough. Nine out of the twenty amino acids cannot be made by the human body, which is why it needs to be supplemented into the diet.

While protein is essential for just about everyone, it is especially important for individuals who plan on staying physically active. Protein is responsible for building new muscle tissue and repairing other tissues. While there is a significant debate on how much protein people need, you can use the general rule of thumb to eat one gram of protein per pound of body weight.

Carbohydrates

On the Ketogenic Diet, you will not have to pay much attention to carbohydrates because they are going to make up such a small part of your diet. It should be noted that there are two general categories of carbohydrates: Complex and Simple.

Simple carbohydrates are sugar molecules that can be digested quickly for an energy boost while complex carbs come from whole-food plants and contain a higher amount of fiber, minerals, and vitamins. When you do eat carbs, these will be the ones that you will want to reach for.

If you wish to calculate the macros to reach your personal goals, I suggest using a calculator online to find your magic numbers. With that in mind, remember that it will be vital that you keep your carb count under 20g in a day. If you are not in ketosis, there is no reason to be following the Ketogenic Diet.

Keto for Women Vs. Men

The truth is, there is a wide variety of people who can benefit from the Ketogenic Diet, whether they are young, old, man, or woman, but the Ketogenic Diet has been known to be especially beneficial for women due to their different hormones and conditions. This diet can be especially beneficial for women who are:

- Lacking results on other diets
- Binge on carbohydrates
- Planning on getting pregnant
- Want a healthy pregnancy
- Struggling with irregular periods
- Struggling with sex hormones
- Going through menopause

Reaching Ketosis

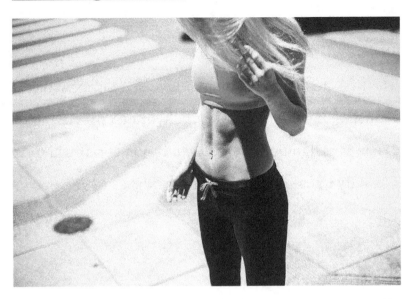

While you are following the Ketogenic Diet, being in Ketosis is going to be the key to your success. Ketosis is a natural state of your metabolic process. Once you have the ability to reach ketosis, this is when your body is going to begin burning the fat you have been storing instead of glucose.

When this process begins, there will be acids that will begin building up in your blood that are known as ketones. Luckily, ketones leave the body in your urine, but it will be important to keep track of the ketones in your body, as they can reach somewhat dangerous levels.

As a beginner, what you may not realize is that achieving ketosis is not as easy as it sounds. Below, you will find some ways to help you get into ketosis and stay there for the most benefit on your new diet!

1. Reduce Carbohydrate Intake

   The first step you are going to take on your new diet is reducing the number of carbohydrates in your diet. When you significantly reduce this number, it will force the body to use fat as energy rather than sugar. As noted earlier, the initial goal should be 20 grams per day or even less, if possible.

2. Increase Healthy Fat

   As you learn how to reduce the number of carbs in your diet, you will want to replace those calories with healthy fats. Remember that your diet is now going to be 70% fat, but it needs to be the right type of fat. Some healthy sources to start out with will be avocados, olive oil, and coconut oil!

3. Test Your Levels

   After you have been following the diet for a few days, you will want to keep a close eye on your ketone levels. The best way to do this is by monitoring your levels with a test. Some of the popular versions include blood tests, breath tests, and urine tests. Each one of these are readily available at the store and should be taken on a daily basis. When you have an exact number, this could help you track what is kicking you out of ketosis.

4. Intermittent Fasting

   A prevalent practice on the Ketogenic Diet is intermittent fasting. While there are several ways to fast, you should speak with your doctor before completing a fast. In controlled cases, you should only fast for a period of ten to fifteen hours. When you go without food for a period of time, this could help put you into ketosis.

5. Physical Exercise

   If all else fails, you can always attempt increasing your physical activity. When you exercise, this will help deplete the glycogen stores you already have in your body. In most cases, these stores would be replenished with carbs, but on the Ketogenic Diet, your body will have no choice but to make the switch.

Signs You Are in Ketosis

As your body begins to undergo the biological adaption of ketosis, this will automatically trigger the reduction of your insulin levels and will increase your fat breakdowns. However, it can be hard to know if you are in ketosis or not. Luckily, there are several signs and symptoms that can tell you whether you are in ketosis or not!

Bad Breath

One of the most common symptoms that are reported on the Ketogenic Diet is bad breath! Bad breath is generally caused by elevated ketone levels, specifically the acetone that is exiting your body through breath and urine.

While this may be not so ideal for your social life, it is an excellent sign that you have reached ketosis! To help resolve this issue, you will want to consider sugar-free gum or just brushing your teeth a few more times a day.

Appetite Suppression

Another side effect of ketosis is appetite suppression. Many individuals have reported that they have decreased hunger while following their new diet. It is believed that this may be due to the increased vegetables and proteins, keeping you fuller for a more extended amount of time! It is possible that ketones also may affect the brain and reduce appetite.

Weight Loss

While following the Ketogenic Diet, you can expect weight loss, even in the first week! While, of course, this is primarily the water and carbs that have been stored in your body, it is just the beginning! Luckily, the Keto diet is known for both long-term and short-term weight loss.

Increased Ketones

As mentioned earlier, you will want to keep track of your ketones. The most reliable method of measuring these ketones is going to be using a blood meter, but you can also use a breath analyzer or urine strip. No matter which method you choose, you will notice an increase in ketones when your body is in ketosis.

Short Term Fatigue

A well-known side effect of the Ketogenic Diet is short-term fatigue. Remember that you are going to be switching the way your body runs, so this is an entirely natural side effect. As you probably expect, any switch you make is not going to happen overnight. In general, it takes people anywhere from seven to thirty days before they reach full ketosis. During this time, you will most likely experience some less than ideal side effects known as the Keto-Flu; we will cover everything you need to know about that in the next chapter. You will want to pay close attention here!

How to Create a Meal Plan

While building your knowledge of the Ketogenic Diet is important, it is just as important to come up with a plan for yourself! When you take the time to make a plan, it leaves less room for failure. As you learn how to follow a meal plan, you will never find yourself with an empty kitchen or, worse, a kitchen with temptations!

Luckily for you, it is easy enough to make your own meal plans, even if you have no idea what you are doing! If you are a true beginner, I suggest only planning one or two meals. As you become more comfortable with your diet and the foods you will be able to enjoy, you can build from that point.

Breakfast

The morning can be a tough time for people, especially when you are trying to get ready and have breakfast at the same time! When you have breakfast prepped already, it will make your life a million times earlier.

For breakfast, you will want to take some of the breakfast options provided them and batch cook them for the week! That way, all you will have to do is decide what you want for breakfast the night before, and you will be set for the morning.

Lunch or Dinner

As far as lunch goes, there is never any reason to go wild and crazy with your choices. All you need is a simple formula to help you create a balanced meal for yourself. The key here is to eat healthily but provide yourself with enough variety to help avoid any boredom. To create a balanced meal, choose one of each from the following list.

- Meat & Cooking Method
- Vegetable & Cooking Method
- Sauce

As long as your kitchen is stocked, you should be able to throw together a keto-friendly meal whenever you need it. Plus, if you make extra for dinner, there is your lunch for the next day! Remember to work smarter, never harder.

Snacks and Dessert

For weight loss purposes, remember that it is a better idea to leave the snacking and sweets behind. But if you are a busy person who is always on the run, it is better to carry snacks with you rather than cheat on your diet because you are in a pinch. Some excellent choices to stock up on could be:

- Pork Rinds
- Meat Sticks

- Dark Chocolate

- Low-carb Nuts

Just like that, you will be prepared for anything that comes your way!

Supplements for Success

When you are first starting the Ketogenic Diet, I suggest trying it for a few weeks on your own. It is going to take some extra effort, but it is absolutely something you can do naturally. If you need a little boost, there are some supplements on the market that can help ease the transition.

Alpha Lipoic Acid and Chromium

If you have issues with your insulin levels, Chromium and r-ALA may be able to help you out. While these two supplements claim to be insulin "mimickers," they actually help increase your sensitivity to insulin to help lower your insulin levels and heighten the glucagon. When this happens, you will get into ketosis quicker.

Hydroxymethylbutyrate (HMB)

This is a popular ketogenic supplement known as BHB salt. It is used as a supplement to minimize the period before you get into ketosis, aka The Keto Flu. HMB is an exogenous ketone, meaning you will be putting synthetic ketone fuel into your body before it naturally makes the change itself. By doing this, it will make the transition time easier.

Carnitine

You probably know this supplement as Acetyl L-Carnitine. This is a popular supplement to use as an energy booster. It seems now that L-Carnitine is actually needed to help boost the formation of ketones in the liver. When you take this supplement, it can help shift your metabolism from glycogen to ketones.

MCT Oil

When you reach ketosis, MCT Oil can be extremely beneficial in keeping you there. This oil has high-quality fats that can give you a quick boost when you need it in your diet. While this doesn't help make your transition more manageable, it will help once you are in ketosis.

Keto Multivitamin

For any people starting a strict kept diet, it can become challenging to get all of your essential fiber, minerals, and vitamins. For this reason, you may want to consider a quality multivitamin. This will help provide you with minerals that are all lost as you transition into ketosis. Either way, you will want to consider taking a supplement that provides you with electrolytes to help you out during the transition process.

Fish Oil

Finally, you will want to consider a supplement of fish oil. Remember that you will need to balance your omega-3s and omega-6s. While Americans generally get twenty times the amount of omega-6 fats they need, a fish oil or cod liver oil will be able to help you create that balance.

While supplements can be beneficial in some cases, they are not necessary. As mentioned earlier, you should give yourself a chance to follow this diet naturally. When you learn how to balance your plate and get your macros just right, you will be able to get into a stay in ketosis with no issue.

Now that you have learned the basics of the Ketogenic Diet, it is time to move onto the next chapter. I want to make sure that you pay close attention here because the Keto-Flu is no joke. It is something that we all go through, but with the tips and tricks provided in the next chapter, you will be able to get through it much easier than I did the first time!

CHAPTER 3: OVERCOMING THE KETO FLU

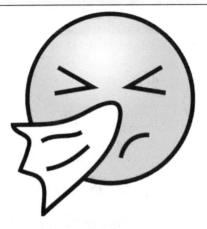

When you first begin the Ketogenic Diet, you are most likely anticipating all of the benefits people mention. While those changes will come at some point, you should be aware of the dreaded Keto Flu. Unfortunately, many people do not anticipate for this metabolic change, and they are unable to push through the potential side effects.

With that in mind, you will want to remember that the Keto flu is only going to be temporary! The fly is most prevalent when the body is attempting to transition into the new, ketogenic state. As soon as your body learns how to be fat-adapted, the symptoms will disappear before you know it!

The first step in tackling the Keto flu is going to be knowing what you are going up against. Luckily, with this book as your handy guide, you will be able to get through the flu with as much grace as possible. You could potentially feel awful, but if you can see the light at the end, you can get through anything. Let's start this chapter off by learning what the Keto flu is.

What Is the Keto Flu?

As you probably could have already guessed, the Keto flu is fairly related to the regular flu. The Keto flu comes about because your metabolism is trying to adjust to running on your new form of energy, fat. This is going to be a drastic change for your body, especially because, for the majority of your life, it has been running off glucose or carbohydrates for energy!

When you begin reducing your carb intake, this is going to begin depleting the glucose stores in your body. This switch can be tough on your body, and from here, you will begin to experience the flu-like symptoms. If you have ever had the flu before, you already know that it is not a great feeling.

Signs & Symptoms of the Keto Flu

So, what can you expect from this infamous Keto Flu? Some of the more common symptoms include:

- Low Energy Levels

- Sugar Cravings

- Lack of Focus

- Inability to Concentrate

- Irritability

- Heart Palpitations

- Insomnia

- Muscle Cramps

- Muscle Soreness

- Constipation

- Diarrhea

- Confusion

- Dizziness

- Nausea

- Stomach Pain

- Overall Brain Fog

If you are starting the Ketogenic Diet for the first time and are nervously awaiting the Keto-Flu, the symptoms listed above will generally start up around the first day or two of your diet. It should be noted that the length and strength of the symptoms are going to vary depending on the person. In fact, some people are lucky enough to skip the Keto flu altogether!

Either way, you can rest assured that the symptoms will only last two weeks, at most. The sooner your body becomes fat-adapted, the better you will feel.

Causes of the Keto Flu

As you expand your knowledge of the Ketogenic Diet, you should be aware that there are four main causes of the keto flu. We will go over each source in detail below to help you lessen the blow of the flu in the first place.

Keto Adaption

Keto adaption is going to be one of the main culprits behind the Keto Flu. The body is incredibly complex and has two primary processes for energy. This includes glycolysis, which is burning glucose for energy and beta-oxidation, which is burning fat for energy. As your body adjusts, you will be switching from one process to the other. This switch is called your metabolic flexibility.

What many people don't realize is that genetics play a major role in our metabolic flexibility. If your metabolic flexibility is low, you are more likely to experience the symptoms of the keto flu. For this reason, some people handle the energy switch easier than others.

Carbohydrate Withdrawal

When you first make the switch to the Ketogenic Diet, you can expect a number of symptoms like cravings for sugar, irritability, and mood swings. There are studies that suggest that our brain is affected by sugar, similar to the way that it is affected by drugs such as cocaine or heroin. When we eat sugar, it releases the "feel good," hormone, dopamine. If you are not getting your "fix," your body is going to protest.

For this reason, when you begin to reduce the number of carbs in your diet, you can expect some of these symptoms. If your diet is currently heavy in refined carbs, sugars, and processed foods, you may have it worse off than others. While this doesn't mean you should jump off the Keto wagon instantly, you should anticipate the flu before it happens.

Lack of Micronutrients

People who first begin the Ketogenic Diet may have a hard time finding the proper balance when it comes to their macronutrients and their micronutrients. I understand that it is difficult enough learning what you can and cannot eat, but these micronutrients are going to be important when it comes to your health.

As you begin the Ketogenic Diet, you already know that you are going to be cutting out a large number of grains, fruits, and vegetables. In order to make up for this, you will need to make sure you are eating a proper amount of keto-friendly foods that will still help you get your micronutrients in. Some of the best foods you can incorporate will be:

- Olive Oil
- Coconut Butter
- Fatty-cut Meat
- Seeds
- Nuts
- Fish
- Asparagus
- Spinach
- Eggplant
- Full-fat dairy

If you find yourself unable to get your micronutrients in, you may want to consider a supplement. Whether it is a multivitamin or a micronutrient powder, you will want to make sure that the item is free from additives, fillers, and sugars. This way, you won't have to worry about non-keto ingredients kicking you out of ketosis.

Electrolyte Imbalance

Last, but definitely not least, we have the electrolyte imbalance. When you begin to make the change of decreasing the number of high carb foods in your diet, you can expect your body to begin losing water at an extremely fast pace.

This happens because the glucose that is stored in your body is bound to anywhere from 2-3 grams of water. As your body begins to adapt, your cells are going to use up the stored glycogen, meaning that the water weight you have been holding onto is going to get flushed out.

When all of this water is flushed out of your system, it is easy to become dehydrated and suffer from an imbalance of electrolytes. Once you become dehydrated, you may experience normal symptoms such as fatigue, headaches, and muscle pain. You will continue to feel this way until you balance your system out again.

For this reason, it will be vital that you are replacing the water and minerals that you are losing during this adaption period. The important minerals you will want to consider include potassium, magnesium, and sodium. By increasing your intake of these minerals, it can help ease your transition period.

The good news is that you will not feel like this forever! These symptoms are only temporary and will reduce as you learn how to put your body into ketosis properly. The even better news is that you can help get rid of the keto flu faster than you thought! Below, you will find some of my favorite tips and tricks of getting rid of the keto flu and jumping into the benefits of the Ketogenic Diet.

How to Get Over the Keto Flu

The anticipation of getting the keto flu can seem overwhelming, but the good news is that you are going to be able to help yourself. The reason people suffer from the keto flu for so long is that they have no idea what is happening to their body! Most people assume that they have to deal with the bad symptoms to get to the benefits of the diet. The truth is, these signs and symptoms from your body are like a cry for help! You don't just feel like junk for no reason! You will want to take the time to listen to your body and see how you can help yourself.

With that in mind, there are several steps you can take to help get you through the keto flu. Below, you will find some of my best tips to help you get over the keto flu and into ketosis with as little misery as possible.

Drink Up and Stay Hydrated

The number one tip I can give you as you begin the ketogenic diet is to stay hydrated! Even if you think that you are drinking enough water, you probably aren't. Staying hydrated should be your top priority as you begin the transition period into ketosis.

As mentioned earlier, water loss is to be expected as you begin your new diet, so these liquids need to be replenished simultaneously. The more often you are drinking, the easier the transition will come. You will see how much drinking water is going to reduce those awful symptoms of nausea, fatigue, and even those wicked headaches.

The best trick up my sleeve to help you drink more water through the day is to keep it in sight! I have a reusable water bottle that is by my side all day long. If you have a visual cue, it acts as an instant reminder to drink more water. I also suggest drinking a majority of the water during the day because it isn't so fun getting up to use the bathroom ten times a night.

Think Electrolytes

While we are on the topic of getting enough water, you will want to keep in mind that balancing your electrolytes is going to be just as important.

Before the ketogenic diet, many people don't have to worry about their electrolytes unless they are highly athletic. As mentioned earlier, your body is about to flush a mass majority of your water weight and electrolytes out of your system during this transition period. With that in mind, it should be noted that people lose electrolytes differently. The good news is that there are several ways for you to mitigate this imbalance.

The first tip I have for you will be increasing your sodium intake! When you increase the sodium in your diet, this could help counterbalance the water loss that is happening in your body. With that in mind, you will want to consider a supplement of Himalayan pink salt rather than the table salt most people have in their house. You would be amazed at the additives found in simple table salt!

Next, you will want to consider eating keto-friendly foods that are rich in potassium. Potassium is in charge of energy production, body temperature, bladder control, heartbeat regulation, and even muscle cramping. If you find yourself having symptoms in any of these areas, you probably need to up your potassium levels. Some of the best sources of this will be pumpkin seeds, mushrooms, and delicious avocado!

Another mineral you will want to make sure you are getting is magnesium. When people have low magnesium levels, this could lead to insulin resistance and depression. To ensure you are getting enough of this micronutrient in your diet, you will want to include food sources like dark chocolate, macadamia nuts, pumpkin seeds, and salmon.

On the Ketogenic Diet, calcium is also going to be important. While most people think that calcium is only important for bone health, it is also vital for your cardiovascular health, muscle contractions, and blood clotting. For this reason, it is a good idea to consume calcium-rich foods like salmon, chia seeds, and leafy greens.

Increase Fats

When your body begins switching over to its new source of energy, you are going to want to make sure that you are providing it with enough fat! Unfortunately, many people are shy about their fat intake when they are first starting their diet because we have been told our whole life that fat is bad! Now that your body is no longer using carbohydrates and sugar as energy, you will need to give your body what it needs!

As you increase your fat consumption while reducing your carb consumption, this will help push your body into using the fat as energy. If you need, you can always supplement with MCT oil to help increase your ketone levels. It is also a good idea to up your fat source and includes foods such as:

- Coconut Oil
- Cacao Butter
- Olive Oil
- Heavy Cream
- Ghee
- Grass-fed Butter
- Avocado Oil
- Bacon Fat
- Walnuts
- Chia Seeds
- Pecans
- Flaxseed
- Fatty Fish
- Sesame Seeds

Work it Out

The next way to help get you over the keto flu will be exercise! This can be hard for some people, especially if they are unable to work through the symptoms provided by the keto flu in the first place. For this reason, I highly suggest light exercise anywhere from two to three times a week.

As you begin moving your body, this will help the switch drastically. As soon as you get over the keto flu, you will be able to resume your normal exercise routine. If you are first starting out, I highly suggest low-intensity exercises. You can try something like yoga, swimming, or even a light walk. With exercise, you will be able to boost your metabolic flexibility and get over the keto flu before you even know it.

Exogenous Ketones

If none of the above work for you, you can always consider exogenous ketones. While your body is attempting to make the switch into ketosis, your body may not be producing enough ketones. For this reason, you may want to add ketone salts or exogenous ketones into your morning routine. By providing your body with what it needs, you can provide your system with ketones before you have even burned through the glycogen stores.

Preventing the Keto Flu

While it is beneficial knowing how to get over the keto flu, it is even better knowing how you can prevent it in the first place! If you are like everyone else in the world, you simply do not have the time to get sick! The good news is that there are some ways that you may be able to skip the keto flu altogether.

Follow the Diet

One of the main reasons beginners fall into the Keto-Flu is due to the fact that they are not following the diet the way they are supposed to! The keto diet best when you are getting the proper micronutrients as well as the right number of macronutrients.

The key to getting to your results is learning how to balance your nutritional needs. Yes, you could hit your macronutrients eating nothing but cottage cheese, but this is a sure way to dive right into the Keto flu. While it is going to be important for you to avoid carbohydrates, you will want to learn how to incorporate plenty of vegetables and seeds to help you get the nutrients you need.

The Power of Sleep

Unfortunately, many people are unaware of how important sleep is for the body. When you are first starting the Ketogenic diet, you will want to get at least seven to eight hours of sleep at night. When you are sleeping more, this could help reduce the fatigue and stress that comes along with the metabolism switch. If you struggle with sleep at night, you may want to consider a couple of power naps during the day!

Supplement

If you feel nothing is working, you can always consider taking a supplement or two. While, of course, you can get everything you need from a balanced diet, some people prefer the ease of a supplement. In the chapter above, you will find a list of some of my favorite supplements to give a try when you need a boost.

CHAPTER 4: BASIC FITNESS FOR THE KETOGENIC DIET

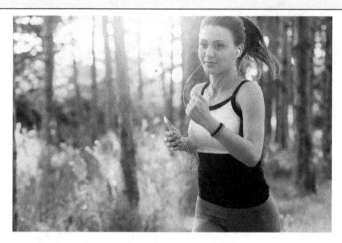

Whether you are following a Ketogenic Diet or not, exercise is almost always beneficial. As you begin to change your diet, you will experience rapid health changes already, but with exercise, you will be able to take your health to a whole new level!

As mentioned earlier, it can be slightly difficult to begin exercise routines when your body is first learning how to get into ketosis. When you are first starting out, you will want to try your best to keep things light but still get your body moving. The question is, how do exercise and the Ketogenic Diet relate?

Ketogenic Diet Impact on Exercise Performance

When you first start the Ketogenic Diet, you will be restricting your carbs. As this process happens, you will be limiting the sugar access for your muscle cells. Once your muscles lack this sugar, they will begin to lose their ability to function at high intensities. For this purpose, high intensities are any activity that can last more than ten seconds.

Due to this process, any activity in the muscle that requires max effort for anywhere from ten seconds to 120 seconds requires sugar. The thing about fat and ketones is that it cannot and never will stand-in for sugar. It is after two minutes of exercise that your body knows how to shift its metabolic pathways and starts burning fat and ketones.

For this reason, you will want to avoid any extreme exercise Some popular examples include

- HIIT (High-Intensity Interval Training)
- Sports such as Lacrosse and Soccer
- Swimming
- Lifting Weights

What to Eat While Exercising on Keto

If you do plan on exercising while on a Ketogenic Diet, it is going to be vital that you get your macronutrients down. Of course, what you eat is going to depend on your goals. Are you looking to gain muscle or lose weight?

Muscle Gain

If you are looking to gain muscle on the Ketogenic Diet, you are going to want to eat more keto-friendly foods. On average, you will want to consider eating anywhere from 250-500 calories extra per day. By doing this, you will be increasing your body weight as well.

Next, most of the calories should be coming from fat. Most athletes put protein as their most important macro, but that isn't true on the Ketogenic Diet. Inf act, your protein intake should only be around one gram of protein per lean body mass that you have. On that note, is carb restriction is impairing your exercise, you may want to consider intermittent fasting.

Fat Loss

When it comes to fat loss, remember that slow loss is still a loss. As you first begin your new diet, you are going to notice weight loss without any exercise, anyway. Generally, you will want to cut down on calories anywhere between 250 and 500 calories. Weight loss comes down to calorie deficit. If you are overweight or obese, you may want to consider a higher calorie deficit.

If you still fail to lose weight after several weeks, consider lower fat intake. That seems counterproductive on the Ketogenic Diet; however, fat is still high in calories. You can still make a majority of your meal's fat-based, but enjoy them in smaller portions.

Cardio on Keto

One of the best options for beginners of the Ketogenic Diet is going to be cardio! Cardio is great for all ages because you don't have to exercise at high-intensities to gain results. As long as you are getting that heart rate up, you will be able to improve your health in a number of different ways.

When you are doing your cardio, you will want to try your best to maintain a moderate intensity. For this, your target heart rate should be 50-80% of your maximum heart rate. For an average 50-year old, your heart rate should be anywhere between 85 and 119 bpm.

Some of my favorite cardio exercises include:

- Aerobics
- Recreational Sports (with Rest Time)

- Light Circuit Training
- Walking
- Cycling

Tips and Tricks for Maximizing Benefits

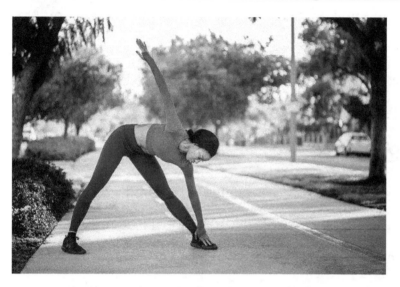

If you do plan on exercising on your diet, the good news is that there are plenty of supplements to help you get to your results quicker and more efficiently. As you pick out your supplements, be sure that they are no-carb. Below, you will find some of my favorite workout supplements.

Creatine

If you are still considering weightlifting on your new diet, you will definitely want to look into purchasing a creatine supplement. This is safe and can enhance your phosphagen system. Generally, you will want to take about five grams a day to help you increase your power, strength, and muscle mass.

Caffeine

Caffeine is very popular among those who exercise on a regular basis. While it can improve exercise performance, it could potentially decrease your ketone production. For this reason, you will want to consider limiting your caffeine intake, but it works when you really need something at the moment.

MCT Oil

As you learned earlier, MCT is a saturated fat that is digested right away. When you need a boost of energy for endurance or cardio, you can always add some MCT oil to your meal before you exercise. Generally, anywhere between one to two tablespoons should do the trick!

Intermittent Fasting

The last trick I have for you before we dive into the recipes is going to be intermittent fasting! You already know what to eat and how to exercise for the most benefit on your new diet, but Intermittent Fasting will help you get max results from the Ketogenic Diet.

Intermittent fasting is a way of eating that helps you cycle between fasting and eating. While many people feel this is a good way to starve yourself, it is actually a way to help you learn self-control when it comes to eating.

We live in a time where food is easily available. We have grocery stores in every town, McDonald's sprinkled everywhere, and a mass majority of people base their day around meals! As you learn to fast, you will be choosing not to eat anywhere between 12-14 hours.

The basic science behind intermittent fasting is to allow your body to use stored energy. When this happens, it will help you burn excess body fat. When we eat, insulin rises and is stored either in the liver or in the muscle. When it comes to carbohydrates, there is very limited storage space, which is where body fat comes from.

If you are interested in Intermittent Fasting, there are several ways to start. Luckily, you can fast for as short or as long as you would like. What is important is that it fits your schedule, and you see benefits from the actions.

Types of Fasting

- **16/8 Method**

This first method is one of the more popular versions of Intermittent Fasting. This one allows an 8-10 hour "eating window" with 14-16 hours of fasting. For the 8-10 hours, you can enjoy two or three meals.

- **5:2 Method**

  Next, we have the 5:2 method. For this version of Intermittent Fasting, you will normally eat for five days of the week, but for the other two, you will only eat about 500-600 calories in the day.

- **Eat-Stop-Eat**

  Another popular method you could try is the Eat-Stop-Eat. This method of intermittent fasting incorporates 24-hour fasts for either one or two times a week. Of course, I highly suggest starting with the other two before trying this one, but it may work best for your schedule at some point!

Now that you understand the basic concepts of the Ketogenic Diet, we can finally get to the good part, eating! In the next few chapters, you will find some of my top favorite recipes. Each recipe is going to be highly nutritious and will help balance your micro and macronutrients on your new diet. Whether you are looking for a healthy breakfast or a quick snack, you will find a recipe for just about any meal!

CHAPTER 5: KETO RECIPES FOR BREAKFAST

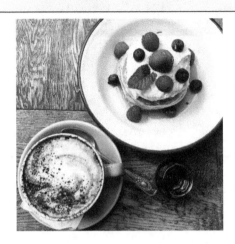

There is nothing quite like starting your morning out with a nice breakfast. The morning is also a great time to get your first boost of fat into your diet and get a boost of energy. Below, you will find some of my favorite, each packed with flavor and nutrition for the Ketogenic Diet.

Spicy Egg Poppers

Yield: Twelve

Time: Forty Minutes

Ingredients

- Eggs [8]
- Cheddar Cheese [1 C.]

- Bacon [10 Strips]

- Jalapeno Peppers [4, Diced]

- Cream Cheese [3 Ounces]

- Salt [Dash]

- Garlic Powder [1 t.]

- Pepper [Dash]

Directions

1. Egg cups are great to have on hand because they are easy to make and easy to grab if you are short on time! To start this recipe, you will first want to prep your stove to 375.

2. Next, you are going to want to take out a cooking pan and place it over a moderate temperature. Once warm, you will cook the bacon for several minutes. You want to make sure that it isn't cooked through so that you can still bend it a bit. When you are finished, save the bacon grease and place it to the side.

3. When you are ready, you will want to take out a bowl and mend the bacon grease with the eggs, cream cheese, and your seasonings. Once this step is complete, set the bowl aside.

4. Now, it is time to assemble the egg cups. The first step of this process is going to be greasing down a muffin tin and carefully line the walls with your bacon. When the bacon is in place, pour in the egg mixture and be sure that you don't overfill it.

5. The final step is going to be sprinkling the cheese over the top of the egg and then gently placing a jalapeno ring on top. When this is complete, pop the dish into the oven for twenty-five minutes and wait.

6. At the end of this time, the egg should look fluffy and slightly browned at the top. If it is cooked to your liking, remove and enjoy your breakfast!

Macros

- ➢ Fats: 25g
- ➢ Carbs: 2g
- ➢ Proteins: 10g

Stuffed Breakfast Pepper

Yield: Four

Time: Forty Minutes

Ingredients

- Bell Pepper [1]

- Spinach [1 C.]
- Onion [.50, Chopped]
- Eggs [2]
- Egg Whites [2]
- Salsa [Optional]
- Pepper [Dash]

Directions

1. These bell peppers are stuffed with flavor and could earn you brownie points for presentation! To start this amazing recipe off, you will first want to prep your stove to 375.

2. As that warms up, take a frying pan and place it over a moderate temperature. When it is warm enough, toss in some olive oil and begin sautéing your onion pieces. If you would like, you can also add in the spinach and salsa for an additional five minutes. When these are cooked to your liking, set them to the side.

3. Next, it is time to get out your baking sheet and line it with tin foil. Once this is complete, carefully slice your bell pepper in half and place the spinach mixture inside of the pepper. With the vegetables placed, you will then

want to carefully spoon in your eggs over the top and then dash some pepper over it.

4. Once the pepper is stuffed, you are going to pop the dish into the oven for half an hour or so. By the end, your eggs should be cooked through and will look fluffy. If they are cooked to your liking, take the dish from the oven and allow them to chill slightly before enjoying.

Macros

- ➢ Fats: 5g
- ➢ Carbs: 2g
- ➢ Proteins: 5g

Keto Breakfast Cookies

Yield: Twelve

Time: Twenty Minutes

Ingredients

- Green Pepper [1, Chopped]
- Onion [.50, Chopped]
- Sausage [5 Oz.]
- Baking Powder [1 t.]
- Almond Flour [1 C.]

- Eggs [3]
- Shredded Cheddar Cheese [1 C.]
- Salt [Dash]

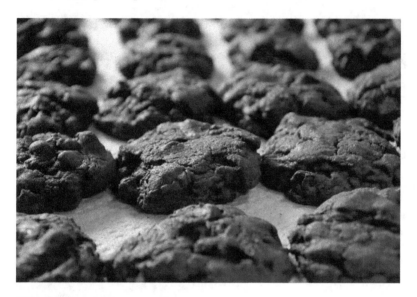

Directions

1. Who wouldn't love to have cookies for breakfast? These breakfast "cookies" offer an excellent boost of fats and proteins to your breakfast while keeping your carb count low. You will want to prepare for this recipe by starting your stove to 375.

2. As this warms up, you can take out your grilling pan and place it over a moderate temperature. Once the pan is heated, add in the peppers, sausage, and the onion

and cook for about five or six minutes. By the end, the vegetables should be soft.

3. When these are prepared, get out a sperate bowl and begin beating the eggs with half of the cheese and the flour, baking powder, and the seasoning. Once the sausage and vegetables have cooled enough, you can also add these in.

4. Now that you are all set to stand line tit without can get out a cooking sheet and line it with a silicone mat or paper. Once this is in place, take your dough and place spoonfuls on the surface. When you are ready, add the rest of the cheese over the top and pop into the oven for ten minutes.

5. At the end of this time, your cookies should be golden and can be removed from the oven. Enjoy your breakfast cookie!

Macros

➤ Fats: 12g

➤ Carbs: 3g

➤ Proteins: 10g

Cream Cheese Breakfast Bombs

Yield: Eight

Time: Thirty Minutes

Ingredients

- Cream Cheese [1 Package]
- Hard-Boiled Eggs [4]
- Bacon [1 Pound]
- Green Onion [2 T.]

Directions

1. Now that you are starting the Ketogenic Diet, I invite you to the incredible world of fat bombs! Fat bombs are incredible to have on hand, whether you want them for breakfast, a quick snack, or even dessert! This recipe is packed with fat and protein to give you that boost of energy you need in the early morning.

2. To begin this recipe, you will want to boil a pot of water so that you can hard boil your eggs. You can finish this task the way you normally would. Once they are cooked through, you can take the shell off and place it to the side to cool a bit.

3. Next, you will want to get out your frying pan and cook your bacon over a moderate temperature until it is nice and crispy. You will want to follow the directions provided on the side of the package to cook the bacon to

your liking. When this step is complete, set the bacon to the side to chill as well.

4. When you are set to make your fat bombs, go ahead and crumble your bacon and chop the hard-boiled egg up into small pieces. Once these items are set, get out the mixing bowl and begin mending the onion, cream cheese, and egg. Once you have your dough, use your hands to roll about eight balls out and place them in the freezer. This will give the balls time to set before rolling them.

5. Now that the balls are slightly hard, you will want to lay your crumbled bacon on a plate and begin rolling the balls in the mixture. You may have to press the ball into the bacon to get it to stick, but don't mush the ball down too much.

6. Finally, your fat bombs are set for your enjoyment!

Macros

➢ Fats: 40g

➢ Carbs: 2g

➢ Proteins: 15g

Cheesy Chive Omelet

Yield: Two

Time: Thirty Minutes

Ingredients

- Eggs [4]
- Cheddar Cheese [1 C.]
- Salt [Dash]
- Butter [1 T.]
- Chives [1 T.]
- Water [.25 C.]
- Pepper [Dash]

Directions

1. As you can tell, eggs are extremely popular on the Ketogenic Diet. They are an excellent source of fat and protein to help out with your macros. Adding cheese in the mix is just the frosting on the cake! When you are ready to make this for breakfast, you will want to take out a frying pan and place it over a moderate temperature. It is important to make sure the surface is hot before doing anything.

2. When the pan is heating up, you will want to combine the water, eggs, and seasoning. Once this is set, carefully pour the mixture into your hot pan and wait several

minutes. You may need to tilt your pan a bit to create an even omelet.

3. After several minutes, go ahead and sprinkle some of the cheese over half of your omelet. Once in place, you will want to use a thin spatula to turn half of the omelet over. This takes practice, but if you are gentle enough, you should be able to complete this task with no issue.

4. For a final touch, you are going to go ahead and sprinkle the rest of the cheese over the top of the omelet and continue to cook until it is browned or cooked to your liking.

5. Finally, sprinkle some pepper and salt over the top for some additional flavor, and then your breakfast is set to be served!

Macros

➤ Fats: 15g

➤ Carbs: 2g

➤ Proteins: 8g

CHAPTER 6: KETO RECIPES FOR LUNCH

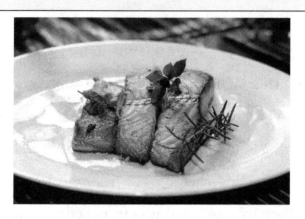

If you are practicing Intermittent Fasting, you will most likely be skipping right to lunch for your first meal. For many people, lunch can be a hard meal to get in because we are at work, at school, or just generally busy. If you plan ahead for lunch, you should have no issues sticking with your diet! Below you will find lunches that are quick and easy to make. Each recipe offers efficient protein and fat to fuel anyone!

Creamy Chicken Salad

Yield: Four

Time: Thirty Minutes

Ingredients

- Chicken Breast [1 Lb.]

- Avocado [2]

- Garlic Cloves [2, Minced]

- Lime Juice [3 T.]

- Onion [.33 C., Minced]

- Jalapeno Pepper [1, Minced]

- Salt [Dash]

- Cilantro [1 T.]

- Pepper [Dash]

Directions

1. If you like traditional chicken salad, this is an excellent alternative to help provide healthier fats along with a good chunk of protein. You will want to start this recipe off my prepping the stove to 400. As this warms up, get out your cooking sheet and line it with paper or foil.

2. Next, it is time to get out the chicken. Go ahead and layer the chicken breast up with some olive oil before seasoning to your liking. I generally use salt and pepper, but feel free to use anything like garlic or onion powder!

3. When the chicken is all set, you will want to line them along the surface of your cooking sheet and pop it into the oven for about twenty minutes. By the end of twenty minutes, the chicken should be cooked through and can

be taken out of the oven for chilling. Once cool enough to handle, you will want to either dice or shred your chicken, dependent upon how you like your chicken salad.

4. Now that your chicken is all cooked, it is time to assemble your salad! You can begin this process by adding everything into a bowl and mashing down the avocado. Once your ingredients are mended to your liking, sprinkle some salt over the top and serve immediately. Whether you like your chicken salad straight out of the bowl or in a low-carb wrap, it can be enjoyed in a number of different ways!

Macros

➢ Fats: 20g

➢ Carbs: 4g

➢ Proteins: 25g

Spicy Keto Chicken Wings

Yield: Four

Time: One Hour

Ingredients

- Chicken Wings [2 Lbs.]

- Cajun Spice [1 t.]

- Smoked Paprika [2 t.]

- Turmeric [.50 t.]

- Salt [Dash]

- Baking Powder [2 t.]

- Pepper [Dash]

Directions

1. When you first begin the Ketogenic Diet, you may find that you won't be eating the traditional foods that may have made up a majority of your diet in the past. While this is a good thing for your health, you may feel you are missing out! The good news is that there are delicious alternatives that aren't lacking in flavor! To start this recipe, you'll want to prep the stove to 400.

2. As this heats up, you will want to take some time to dry your chicken wings with a paper towel. This will help remove any excess moisture and get you some nice, crispy wings!

3. When you are all set, take out a mixing bowl and place all of the seasonings along with the baking powder. If you feel like it, you can adjust the seasoning levels however you would like. Once these are set, go ahead

and throw the chicken wings in and coat evenly. If you have one, you'll want to place the wings on a wire rack that is placed over your baking tray. If not, you can just lay them across the baking sheet.

4. Now that your chicken wings are set, you are going to pop them into the stove for thirty minutes. By the end of this time, the tops of the wings should be crispy. If they are, take them out from the oven and flip them so that you can bake the other side. You will want to cook these for an additional thirty minutes.

5. Finally, take the tray from the oven and allow to cool slightly before serving up your spiced keto wings. For additional flavor, serve with any of your favorite, keto-friendly dipping sauce.

Macros

- ➤ Fats: 7g
- ➤ Carbs: 1g
- ➤ Proteins: 60g

Cilantro and Lime Creamed Chicken

Yield: Four

Time: Thirty Minutes

Ingredients

- Chicken Breast [4 Pieces]

- Red Pepper Flakes [1 t.]

- Cilantro [1 T.]

- Salt [Dash]

- Lime Juice [2 T.]

- Chicken Broth [1 C.]

- Onion [.25 C., Chopped]

- Olive Oil [1 T.]

- Heavy Cream [.50 C.]

- Pepper [Dash]

Directions

1. If you are looking for a dish that is a bit different, this recipe is going to be perfect for you. Between the cilantro and the lime, this dish offers a fresh twist on traditional chicken. Many people feel that in order to lose weight, they need to give up flavor, but on the Ketogenic Diet, that is simply not the case! To begin this recipe, you will want to get out your cooking skillet and place it over a moderate temperature.

2. As the skillet heats, go ahead and season the chicken breast according to your taste. For this particular recipe, you will want to consider using the seasonings provided

in the list above, but feel free to adjust levels to your own taste. Once seasoned to your liking, throw the chicken into the skillet and cook for about eight minutes on each side. When the chicken is cooked through, take it out of the pan and place to the side.

3. Next, you are going to add the onion into the hot pan and cook them for a minute before also adding in the cilantro, pepper flakes, lime juice, and the chicken broth. If you don't have chicken broth on hand, feel free to use water. Once these items are in place, bring to a boil for ten minutes.

4. Last-minute, you are going to whisk in your heavy cream and add in the chicken so that it can be coated in the sauce you just made. For extra flavor, add in some more cilantro, and then your chicken can be served by itself or with a keto-friendly vegetable!

Macros

- ➢ Fats: 20g
- ➢ Carbs: 6g
- ➢ Proteins: 30g

Cheesy Ham Quiche

Yield: Six

Time: Forty Minutes

Ingredients

- Eggs [8]
- Zucchini [1 C., Shredded]
- Heavy Cream [.50 C.]
- Ham [1 C., Diced]
- Mustard [1 t.]
- Salt [Dash]

Directions

1. Unlike traditional quiche, this version is crustless! Because there is no crust, this recipe offers a low-carb option for those who are still looking to make a savory meal for breakfast or lunch. For this recipe, you can start off by prepping your stove to 375 and getting out a pie plate for your quiche.

2. Next, it is time to prep the zucchini. First, you will want to go ahead and shred it into small pieces. Once this is complete, take a paper towel and gently squeeze out the excess moisture. This will help avoid a soggy quiche.

3. When the step from above is complete, you will want to place the zucchini into your pie plate along with the cooked ham pieces and your cheese. Once these items

are in place, you will want to whisk the seasonings, cream, and eggs together before pouring it over the top.

4. Now that your quiche is set, you are going to pop the dish into your stove for about forty minutes. By the end of this time, the egg should be cooked through, and you will be able to insert a knife into the center and have it come out clean.

5. If the quiche is cooked to your liking, take the dish from the oven and allow it to chill slightly before slicing and serving.

Macros

➢ Fats: 25g

➢ Carbs: 2g

➢ Proteins: 20g

Loaded Cauliflower Rice

Yield: Four

Time: Thirty Minutes

Ingredients

- Cauliflower [1 Head]

- Cheddar Cheese [1 C.]

- Bacon [1 Lb.]

- Chives [.50 C.]
- Salt [Dash]

Directions

1. Sometimes, you just want something basic for lunch. This loaded cauliflower rice is fairly easy to make and only requires a handful of ingredients! The first step of this recipe is going to be ricing your cauliflower. You can choose to do this by hand, or you can purchase cauliflower rice in the frozen section.

2. Next, you will want to take several moments to cook your bacon. You can complete this task by heating a grilling pan over a moderate temperature and cook the bacon for four or five minutes on either side. I like my bacon crispy, but that is completely up to you!

3. When you are set, you are going to place your cauliflower rice into a microwave-safe bowl and sprinkle your shredded cheese over the top. When this is set, go ahead and pop the bowl into the microwave for a minute and allow for the rice to cook through and the cheese to melt.

4. Once the step from above is complete, top the dish off with your bacon pieces and season to your liking. Just like that, lunch will be ready for you!

Macros

➢ Fats: 10g

➢ Carbs: 5g

➢ Proteins: 5g

CHAPTER 7: KETO RECIPES FOR DINNER

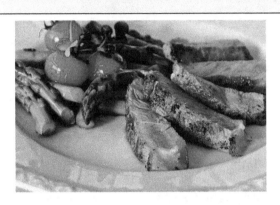

Dinner is a very important meal for the day. Whether you are cooking for one or cooking for your whole family, dinner can truly bring people together. Hopefully, at this point in your day, you will be able to take some time to slow down and enjoy the process of cooking. If not, there are plenty of recipes that are still quick and easy to make — the recipes to follow range for a variety of flavors for just about anyone.

Buttery Garlic Steak

Yield: Four

Time: Thirty Minutes

Ingredients

- Steak [1 Lb.]
- Grass-fed Butter [5 T.]

- Garlic Cloves [5 T., Minced]
- Parsley [.25 C.]
- Salt [Dash]

Directions

1. One of the secret tips I can give you for the Ketogenic Diet is to put butter on absolutely everything that you can. Vegetable? Butter. Side dish? Butter. Main dish? Butter! This garlic butter steak is out of this world and incredibly easy to make. Before you even think about cooking, you will want to set aside several moments to season your steak properly. The best technique to use would be patting the steak down and then season with pepper and salt on both sides. Be generous with your seasoning!

2. Next, it is time to cook your steak. If you have a heavy-duty skillet, use it! Once you have your skillet, bring it over a moderate temperature and heat for several minutes without anything in it. Once hot, add in the steak and sear both sides for about three minutes. If you like your steak cooked past medium-rare, leave it on longer. When the steak is cooked to your liking, remove it from the pan and set to the side.

3. Now that your steak is cooked through, it is time to make the garlic butter. To accomplish this, you will want to lower the heat in your skillet and begin melting your butter. Once the butter has been liquified, you will next add in the garlic and cook for an additional minute. When the garlic turns a golden color, take the pan away from the heat.

4. The next step will be slicing up your steak. Once it is complete, carefully drizzle your butter sauce over the top until the steak becomes completely coated. As a final touch, garnish with some fresh parsley and enjoy your dinner.

Macros

> Fats: 25g

> Carbs: 2g

> Proteins: 25g

Baked Lemon Salmon

Yield: Four

Time: Twenty Minutes

Ingredients

- Salmon [4 Pieces]

- Salt [Dash]
- Lemon Juice [2 T.]
- Lemon [1]
- Grass-fed Butter [2 T.]
- Pepper [Dash]

Directions

1. If you enjoy your fresh seafood, this lemon salmon fillet is going to blow your mind. The lemon offers a refreshing twist to the fish and goes perfect with a side of cauliflower or broccoli. To start this recipe off, you will first want to go ahead and prep the stove to 400. As it heats up, get out your baking sheet and line it.

2. When you are set to cook the fish, you will first want to run it under water before patting it down with some paper towels. Once this has been done, place the fish with the skin side facing down.

3. Next, you will melt your butter and carefully spoon it over each piece of fish. With the butter in place, you can season with some pepper and salt according to your own taste.

4. Now that the fish has been seasoned, you will then want to pour your lemon juice over the top and place a slice of lemon on top of each salmon filet.

5. When you are ready to cook your meal, you are now going to pop the dish into the stove for fifteen minutes. By the end of this time, you will know that your fish is cooked through if you can flake it easily with a fork. If it is cooked through, take the dish out from the oven and allow it to chill for several minutes.

6. Finally, serve the fish with your favorite keto-friendly side, and enjoy your meal.

Macros

➢ Fats: 20g

➢ Carbs: 3g

➢ Proteins: 20g

One Sheet Fajitas

Yield: Six

Time: Twenty Minutes

Ingredients

- Chicken Breast [1 Lb.]

- Fajita Seasoning [2 T.]

- Cilantro [.25 C.]

- Onion [1, Sliced]

- Red Bell Pepper [1, Sliced]

- Green Bell Pepper [1, Sliced]

- Olive Oil [3 T.]

- Salt [Dash]

- Lime Juice [2 T.]

Directions

1. What is better than fajitas for dinner? Fajitas that you can make using one pan! This recipe is easy to make and easy to enjoy. To begin, you will want to go ahead and prep the oven to 400. As this warms up, you can also get out the one baking sheet it is going to take for this recipe.

2. When you are all set, you will want to throw all of the ingredients from above into a mixing bowl and season with the pepper, salt, and the lime juice. Once this is set, spread the items across your baking sheet as evenly as possible.

3. Now that your sheet is set, you are going to pop it into the stove for twenty minutes. By the end of this time, the chicken should be cooked through. If you like

everything a little crispy, you can go ahead and broil the ingredients for an additional two minutes.

4. When your meal is set, take it out from the stove and allow it to chill for two minutes. As a final touch, season with some fresh cilantro and enjoy your keto-friendly fajitas!

Macros

- ➢ Fats: 10g
- ➢ Carbs: 4g
- ➢ Proteins: 25g

Balsamic Chicken

Yield: Four

Time: One Hour

Ingredients

- Chicken Breast [4 Pieces]
- Grass-fed Butter [2 T.]
- Salt [Dash]
- Roasted Garlic Cloves [4]
- Mushrooms [2 C., Sliced]
- Thyme [1 t.]
- Chives [1 T.]

- Red Pepper Flakes [1 t.]
- Balsamic Vinegar [.25 C.]
- Water [.50 C.]
- Onions [.25 C., Chopped]

Directions

1. While following the Ketogenic Diet, it is a good idea to always have chicken on hand. This is a very versatile item and can offer a pack of protein as long as it is paired with the proper fats to balance out your diet. While this recipe does take a bit longer, the flavor will be worth the wait. You can begin this recipe by prepping the stove to 350 and getting out your baking sheet.

2. As the stove warms up, you will want to take out your skillet and begin heating the butter in it. Once the butter is melted, add in the chicken pieces and season with your pepper and salt. When the meat is seasoned to your liking, grill each side of the chicken for three or four minutes. Once the chicken is cooked through, place it onto your baking sheet, and cook in your heated stove for an additional twenty-five minutes.

3. As the chicken cooks, you will want to melt some more butter in your heated pan. Once melted, add in your mushrooms and onions. You will want to sauté these items for a minute before adding in the roasted garlic, thyme, red pepper flakes, and the balsamic vinegar. After these ingredients have cooked for a minute, pour in the water and stir until the liquid begins to reduce.

4. Finally, you are going to pour the mixture over your chicken and serve the dish hot. If you would like, you can serve with fresh parsley or chopped chives for some nice additional flavors.

Macros

➢ Fats: 15g

➢ Carbs: 8g

➢ Proteins: 30g

Cheesy Keto Meatballs

Yield: Three

Time: Twenty Minutes

Ingredients

- Ground Beef [1 Lb.]

- Salt [Dash]

- Garlic Powder [1 t.]
- Parmesan Cheese [3 T.]
- Mozzarella Cheese [1 C.]
- Pepper [Dash]

Directions

1. Whether you are looking for a snack to pop into your mouth quickly or a delicious meal, this recipe can help you out. While meatballs are delicious by themselves, imagine stuffing them with cheese. To begin this recipe, you will want to take some time to chop your fresh mozzarella into bite-sized pieces.

2. When this first step is complete, season the ground beef to your liking and then carefully wrap each cheese piece with the ground beef and begin creating your meatballs. This recipe should make between nine and ten balls.

3. Once you are set to cook your meal, you will want to take out your frying pan and place it over a moderate temperature. When the pan is warm, you can go ahead and grill the meatballs on all sides for five minutes or so. By the end of this time, the meatballs should be crispy and can be served over some zoodles or enjoyed by themselves!

Macros

- ➤ Fats: 35g
- ➤ Carbs: 2g
- ➤ Proteins: 40g

CHAPTER 8: KETO SALAD RECIPES

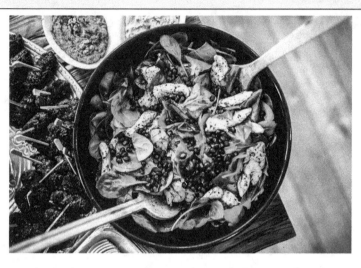

For a quick and easy meal, it is a great idea to have salads on hand. These can be staples in your diet, whether you are eating salad for lunch or dinner. If you incorporate any of these meals throughout the week, it can help you save time and stick to your diet on the busiest of days.

Pesto Chicken Salad

Yield: Four

Time: Thirty Minutes

Ingredients

- Chicken Breast [4 Pieces]

- Pesto [.50 C.]

- Cherry Tomatoes [1 C.]

- Spinach [3 C.]
- Salt [Dash]
- Olive Oil [3 T.]

Directions

1. For another alternative for plain old, baked chicken, you will want to consider this delicious Pesto chicken salad! To start off, you are going to want to go ahead and prep the stove to 350. As this warms up, place your chicken pieces onto a baking plate and coat with the pepper, salt, and olive oil. When this is done, pop the dish into the oven for forty minutes.

2. When the chicken is cooked through and no longer pink on the inside, you will now take it away from the oven and cool slightly before handling.

3. Once you can handle the chick, you will want to toss it into a bowl along with the pesto and your sliced tomatoes. When the ingredients are mended to your liking, place over a bowl of fresh spinach and enjoy your salad.

Macros

➤ Fats: 12g
➤ Carbs: 2g

> Proteins: 40g

Fresh Summer Salad

Yield: Four

Time: Ten Minutes

Ingredients

- Olive Oil [2 T.]
- Thyme [1 t.]
- Oregano [1 t.]
- Ricotta Cheese [.25 C.]
- Basil [1 Leaf, Chopped]
- Balsamic Vinegar [1 T.]
- Cucumber [1, Sliced]
- Tomato [3, Sliced]
- Radishes [5, Sliced]
- Onion [1, Sliced]

Directions

1. Don't be fooled by the name; this salad can be enjoyed at any time of the year! If you are looking for a meatless dish, this is the perfect recipe for you! The first step you will want to take for this recipe will be making your ricotta cheese. You can complete this in a small bowl by

mending the thyme, oregano, basil in with the ricotta cheese.

2. Next, you will be making your own dressing! For this task, all you have to do is whisk your vinegar and olive oil together. Once this is complete, season however you would like.

3. Finally, take some time to slice and dice the vegetables according to the directions above. When your veggies are all set, you will want to assemble them in your serving dishes and pour the dressing generously over the top. As a final touch, dollop your ricotta cheese over your salad, and then your salad will be ready for serving.

Macros

➤ Fats: 10g

➤ Carbs: 8g

➤ Proteins: 5g

Keto Taco Salad

Yield: Six

Time: Twenty Minutes

Ingredients

- Ground Beef [1 Ln.]

- Olive Oil [3 T.]

- Pepper [Dash]

- Onion Powder [1 T.]

- Cumin [1 T.]

- Garlic Clove [1 T., Minced]

- Tomato [1, Chopped]

- Sour Cream [.50 C.]

- Black Olives [.50 C.]

- Cheddar Cheese [.25 C.]

- Cilantro [2 T.]

- Green Pepper [1, Chopped]

Directions

1. With taco salad, you will be able to enjoy everything that you love about tacos with a lot less carbohydrates! Whether you prepare this for taco Tuesday or a quick lunch, it is sure to be a crowd-pleaser!

2. Start this recipe off by taking out your grilling pan and place it over a moderate temperature. As it warms up, you can add in the olive oil and let that sizzle. When you are set, add in the green pepper, spices, and ground beef. You can also use ground turkey in this recipe if

that is more your style. Go ahead and cook these ingredients together for ten minutes or so.

3. When you are all set, place some mixed greens into a bowl and cover with the meat mixture you just created. If you would like some extra flavor, sprinkle some cheddar cheese over the top along with some sour cream.

Macros

- ➢ Fats: 20g
- ➢ Carbs: 5g
- ➢ Proteins: 20g

Mixed Vegetable Tuna Salad

Yield: Four

Time: Ten Minutes

Ingredients

- Canned Tuna [1 Can]
- Olive Oil [2 T.]
- Parsley [.25 C.]
- Red Pepper [1, Roasted & Chopped]
- Artichoke Hearts [.50 C., Diced]
- Black Olives [.25 C.]

- Basil [2 T.]
- Lemon Juice [2 T.}
- Pepper [Dash]

Directions

1. When you are in a rush, you can't go wrong with tuna salad! To save yourself even more time, you can go ahead and prep this tuna salad at the beginning of the week so that all you will have to do is grab and go!

2. For this recipe, get out a mixing bowl and mend all of the items from the list above. Once combined, feel free to season with pepper and salt to your liking.

3. For serving purposes, this tuna salad can be enjoyed in a number of different ways. You can eat it right out of the bowl, scooped into a lettuce wrap, or served over a bed of salad!

Macros

- Fats: 15g
- Carbs: 3g
- Proteins: 10g

Lemon Shrimp Salad

Yield: Four

Time: Twenty Minutes

Ingredients

- Mixed Greens [5 C.]
- Olive Oil [2 T.]
- Shrimp [1 Lb.]
- Sliced Almonds [.25 C.]
- Avocado [2, Sliced]
- Pepper [Dash]
- Lemon Juice [2 T.]

Directions

1. When people think about making a salad for lunch, they often think of either chicken or steak over the top. Have you ever considered shrimp on your salad? It is an awesome alternative when you don't feel like having chicken or steak again. To begin this recipe, you will first need to sear your shrimp.

2. For some added flavor, go ahead and mix your shrimp with some pepper and lemon juice. When it is coated to your liking, you are going to place it into a grilling pan over a moderate temperature. We are only going to sear the shrimp so it should only take two to three minutes

on either side. You will just want to make sure that the shrimp is cooked thoroughly.

3. When the shrimp is cooked to your liking, it is time to assemble your salad. Go ahead and place your mixed greens into your serving bowls and squeeze some lemon juice over the top. Once these items are in place, add in the olive oil and begin layering the avocado on top.

4. For a final touch, add in the shrimp and sliced almonds for a bit of a crunch. Just like that, your salad will be fresh and ready for serving.

Macros

➢ Fats: 30g

➢ Carbs: 10g

➢ Proteins: 30g

CHAPTER 9: KETO RECIPES FOR SNACKS

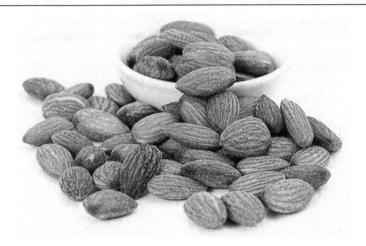

As you begin the Ketogenic Diet, you may find it surprising, but many people find that their meals are filling enough that they don't need a snack in the first place! However, if you are going to snack, you will want to make sure that it is Keto-friendly.

In this chapter, you will find some quick and easy keto snacks to help you get started. Keep in mind that if you are looking to lose weight on your new diet, you will need to keep your calories and snacking to a minimum. You may find that you are hungry to begin with, but it will get better with time!

Sweet Cinnamon Roll Fat Bomb

Yield: Twenty

Time: Ten Minutes

Ingredients

- Cream Cheese [1 Package]
- Stevia [.25 C.]
- Grass-fed Butter [.50 C.]
- Heavy Whipping Cream [3 T.]
- Vanilla Extract [.25 t.]
- Stevia [2 T.]
- Ground Cinnamon {2 t.]
- Almond Flour [1 C.]
- Cream Cheese [1 Oz.]

Directions

1. When you are first starting the Ketogenic Diet, it is a good idea to always have fat bombs on hand. If you are experiencing symptoms from the Keto-Flu or are just feeling a little tired, a fat bomb should be able to pick you right up!

2. You will begin this recipe by making the balls. In order to do this, you will want to soften your first package of

cream cheese and mend it in a bowl with your softened butter. Once these are combined well, you can add in the vanilla extract.

3. Next, you will add in your ground cinnamon and flour. Now that you have your dough, you will want to use your hands to create balls. Generally, you should be able to make anywhere between fifteen and twenty fat bombs. When this step is complete, pop the dish into your freezer for thirty minutes so that they can set.

4. Your next step is going to be making your frosting. You can complete this task by combining the vanilla extract with your heavy whipping cream, cream cheese, and a touch of sweetener.

5. When your balls are solid enough, remove from the freezer and place onto your counter. Here, you can begin to drizzle or dunk the balls into your frosting and then put back into the freezer.

6. After an additional ten minutes or so, your snack will be set for your enjoyment!

Macros

➢ Fats: 15g

➢ Carbs: 1g

> Proteins: 2g

Sausage and Cheese Puffs

Yield: Four

Time: Thirty Minutes

Ingredients

- Butter [4 T., Melted]
- Cheddar Cheese [2 C.]
- Sausage [1 Lb.]
- Eggs [4}
- Garlic Powder [.25 t.]
- Baking Powder [.25 t.]
- Coconut Flour [.25 C.]
- Sour Cream [3 T.]
- Salt [Dash]

Directions

1. For another quick and easy snack, you will want to try these little balls of heaven! They are soft, fluffy, and offer a good chunk of fat when you need it! This recipe can be used as a snack or can be an excellent addition to breakfast as well! To start off, you will want to prep the

stove to 375. You can also get out a baking sheet; you are going to need it later.

2. Next, it is time to get out the griddle! Go ahead and bring it over a moderate temperature. As it warms up, place your butter and let it melt. Once it is melted, add in your sausage and cook on both sides. Generally, this should only take three or four minutes. When it is cooked to your liking, take it out from the pan and set to the side.

3. Your next step will require a mixing bowl. Once you have your bowl, mend together the garlic, salt, sour cream, eggs, and four tablespoons of melted butter. When these are combined, add in the baking powder and coconut flour. Now that your dough is created, you will also want to fold in the cooked sausage and your shredded cheese.

4. Next, you will want to take your hands and make balls of batter. As you do this, line them up evenly across the surface of your baking sheet. When this is set, pop the dish into the stove for twenty minutes. By the end, the balls should be browned and cooked through.

5. If they are cooked to your liking, take the dish from the stove and chill slightly before digging into your snack.

Macros

- ➢ Fats: 50g

- ➢ Carbs: 2g

- ➢ Proteins: 30g

<u>Frozen Berry Bites</u>

Yield: Four

Time: Three Hours

Ingredients

- Milk [2 T.]

- Full-fat Yogurt [2 C.]

- Blackberries [.25 C.]

- Raspberries [.25 C.]

- Stevia [1 Packet]

Directions

1. As you learned in the second chapter, fruit is generally left out of the Ketogenic Diet because it is high in sugar and carbs. However, sometimes it is nice to have as a treat! You will note that this recipe is slightly higher in carbohydrates, but as long as you count it with your

macros, you can still enjoy some frozen berry bites in moderation!

2. To begin this recipe, you will first want to take some time to mash down the fruit into smaller pieces. When this is complete, you can add in your milk and yogurt. Once in place, combine everything together as well as possible so that the fruit is spread evenly.

3. When you are set, pour the mixture into an ice cube tray and pop into the freezer for about three hours. By the end, you can pop out the chunks, and your berry bites will be set for snack time.

Macros

➢ Fats: 5g

➢ Carbs: 7g

➢ Proteins: 5g

Cream Cheese and Ham Rolls

Yield: Four

Time: Five Minutes

Ingredients

- Dill Pickles [15]

- Cream Cheese [1 Package]

- Sliced Ham [15 Slices]

Directions

1. When you need a quick snack, this is the perfect recipe to whip together. Plus, finger foods can be a lot of fun if you are trying to get a child or friend to try out the Ketogenic Diet!

2. To make this quick and easy snack, you will first want to lay out each slice of ham in front of you. When this is done, carefully spread about a tablespoon of cream cheese across the surface. You will want to do this carefully because the ham can tear easily if the slices are not thick enough.

3. Finally, you are going to place one small pickle into the center and roll it up tightly. If needed, you can use a toothpick to keep your rolls in place.

4. When the step from above is complete, pop the dish into the fridge for at least two hours before serving.

Macros

➢ Fats: 30g

➢ Carbs: 6g

➢ Proteins: 20g

Keto-friendly Crackers

Yield: Twenty-five

Time: Twenty Minutes

Ingredients

- Almond Flour [2 C.]
- Eggs [2]
- Grass-fed Butter [8 T., Soft]
- Salt [Dash]

Directions

1. While these crackers don't particularly offer a high amount of fat or protein, this recipe is great to have on hand. Crackers are versatile, whether you are looking for a snack or something on the side. You will find that many crackers in the market are filled with additives and high in carbs. To help keep them keto-friendly, you can make your own! To start out, prep the stove to 350 and get out your favorite baking sheet.

2. When you are set, take out a bowl and mend together the almond flour with the softened butter. For this step, it can be extremely helpful to have a hand mixer!

3. Once these two items are blended together, add in your eggs one at a time and punch some salt over the top. You will want to continue stirring these items until you get a perfectly smooth dough.

4. Next, you will want to place the dough in between two pieces of parchment paper and begin rolling out the dough onto your baking sheet. By doing this, you can make sure that the dough is flat and even. You will want to roll the dough out until it is about an eighth of an inch in thickness.

5. When you are done rolling the dough, use a pizza cutter to score your dough. You can make the crackers as big or as small as you would like! Once you have cut the dough up, pop the dish into the stove for fifteen minutes. By the end, the crackers should be golden.

6. As a final touch, sprinkle some more salt over the top, and then your crackers will be all ready for you to enjoy!

Macros

➢ Fats: 10g

➢ Carbs: 1g

➢ Proteins: 2g

CHAPTER 10: KETO RECIPES FOR DESSERT

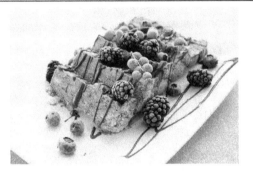

Last but not least, we will end this book on the sweetest part of the day, dessert! While other diets normally discourage anything sweet or along the lines of dessert, you will be able to enjoy keto-friendly desserts on your new diet!

Much like with snacking, you will want to consider keeping dessert to a minimum if you are looking to lose weight on your diet. Remember that the only way you are going to lose weight is if you have a calorie deficit. For this reason, I suggest only indulging in dessert once or twice a week. If you have the macros left for it, I say go for it!

Chocolate Peanut Butter Bombs

Yield: Ten

Time: Five Minutes

Ingredients

- Almond Flour [2 T.]

- Stevia [2 T.]

- Vanilla Extract [.25 t.]

- Olive Oil [1 T.]

- Peanut Butter [.25 C.]

- Chocolate Chips [.50 C.]

Directions

1. Is there a better combination than peanut butter and chocolate? When you put these two things together, you will have a delicious and keto-friendly dessert ready when you need it. To start out, you will want to get out your mixing bowl so that you can mend the flour, sweetener, peanut butter, and vanilla extract. From this, you will get your dough.

2. When you are all set, you can use your hands to roll balls from this mixture. With this recipe, you should be able to make between ten and twelve balls. Once these are set, you will want to place them on a plate and pop into the freezer for half an hour.

3. After the balls have set and are on the harder side, remove from the freezer and place back onto the

counter. Now, you will want to carefully melt your chocolate chips in a microwave-safe bowl. Generally, this will only take thirty to forty seconds. Make sure you watch the chocolate chips because they can burn fairly easily.

4. Once the chocolate has been melted, carefully dip each ball into the melted chocolate and coat evenly. If you would like, you can also drizzle the chocolate over the top. Once you have put the chocolate on the balls, you will want to place the plate of balls back into the freezer for an additional fifteen minutes.

5. Once this time has passed, the chocolate peanut butter balls will be ready for dessert! Enjoy!

Macros

➤ Fats: 5g

➤ Carbs: 1g

➤ Proteins: 3g

Keto Ice Cream

Yield: Ten

Time: Thirty Minutes

Ingredients

- Egg Yolks [2]
- Creamy Peanut Butter [.50 C.]
- Heavy Whipping Cream [2 C.]
- Cocoa Powder, Unsweetened [2 T.]
- Erythritol [.50 C.]

Directions

1. When you first start the Ketogenic Diet, you will quickly learn that all of your favorite foods are going to be high in carbs, high in added sugar, and filled with additives that are bad for your health. Luckily, you will be able to make a majority of your favorites all on your own! Here, we have a simple chocolate and peanut butter ice cream that only requires five ingredients!

2. The first step of making your own ice cream will be taking out a mixing bowl and dissolving your cocoa powder. For this, you will only need about two tablespoons of water. When this is set, place it into a food processor with the rest of the ingredients and mend everything together for a few seconds.

3. When this is set, you are going to pour the mixture into a bowl and freeze for around three hours. After this, you will have delicious ice cream that is still keto-friendly! If

you have an ice cream maker, you can also pour the mixture into here and have ice cream almost in an instant!

Macros

- ➢ Fats: 30g
- ➢ Carbs: 4g
- ➢ Proteins: 5g

Cheesecake Fat Bombs

Yield: Fifteen

Time: Thirty Minutes

Ingredients

- Fresh Raspberries [.25 C.]
- Cream Cheese [1 Package]
- Stevia [2 T.]
- Grass-fed Butter [3 T.]
- Vanilla Extract [1 T.]

Directions

1. If you are a fan of cheesecake, you are going to absolutely love this recipe. By making these fat bombs, it is a great way to eat your cheesecake guilt-free because it is keto-friendly! Though it is delicious, remember to

keep your dessert in moderation! Calories still count as calories, and there is such thing as too much fat on the Ketogenic Diet. You have to find the balance while still enjoying your treats.

2. To start this recipe, you will want to take some time to mash your raspberries down into smaller bits. Once the raspberry has been smashed, add in the cream cheese and the butter. To make this easier, you can leave the cream cheese and butter out at room temperature for around an hour or so.

3. Now that you have your mixture take your hands to create balls from the dough and place it into your freezer for thirty minutes. At the end of this time, your fat bombs will be solid and set for dessert.

Macros

➢ Fats: 10g

➢ Carbs: 1g

➢ Proteins: 2g

Lemon Bars

Yield: Eight

Time: One Hour

Ingredients

- Almond Flour [2 C.]
- Lemons [2]
- Eggs [3]
- Erythritol [1 C.]
- Butter [.25 C.]

Directions

1. Not everyone is a chocolate lover, and that is okay to admit! These lemon bars are dense and fluffy. If you need something to bring to a party, this is the perfect recipe to try out! You don't have to be following a Ketogenic Diet to enjoy this one.

2. You will want to start this recipe off by prepping the stove to 350. As the stove heats up, line your baking dish with some paper and begin mixing together the almond flour with the erythritol. For a touch more of flavor, feel free to add a pinch of salt.

3. When you are set, pour the mixture into your baking dish and pop it into the stove for twenty minutes. By the end of this time, the bars should be set and can be taken out of the oven.

4. Next, it is time to make the lemon zest for your bars! In a bowl, you will want to juice the two lemons and add the

zest from one. When these are set, mix in your eggs along with a cup of erythritol and another cup of your almond flour. Once this step is complete, pour it onto the crust and pop the dish back into the stove for an additional twenty-five minutes.

5. When your bars are cooked to your liking, take the dish from the oven and allow it to chill for ten minutes before slicing the bars up. For a finishing touch, sprinkle some more erythritol over the top and even decorate with a slice of lemon!

Macros

- ➢ Fats: 25g
- ➢ Carbs: 5g
- ➢ Proteins: 7g

Ketogenic Cookie Dough

Yield: Four

Time: Ten Minutes

Ingredients

- Cream Cheese [1 Package]
- Dark Chocolate Chips [.25 C.]
- Grass-fed Butter [2 T.]

- Vanilla Extract [1 T.]

- Creamy Peanut Butter [5 T.]

- Stevia [.25 C.]

Directions

1. We are all guilty of eating raw cookie dough. Now, you can enjoy raw cookie dough on purpose, while still following your diet! This is another version of a fat bomb, meaning you can enjoy it as a dessert or make other people extremely jealous of your delicious snack!

2. To make these fat bombs, you are going to take all of the ingredients from the list above, minus the chocolate chips, and place them into your food processor. Once you have created your dough, you will next fold in your chocolate chips.

3. When this step is complete, use your hands to create small balls from the dough. As you do this, you will want to place each ball onto a plate so that you can place the plate into the freezer for thirty minutes.

4. After this time has passed, you will have fat bombs for dessert! Enjoy!

Macros

➢ Fats: 20g

- ➢ Carbs: 6g
- ➢ Proteins: 5g

CHAPTER 11: THE SOLUTION TO YOUR WEIGHT PROBLEMS

Routines are very important on this diet, and it's something that will help you stay healthy. As such, in this phase, we are going to be giving you tips and tricks to make this diet work better for you and help you get an idea of routines that you can put in place for yourself.

Tip number one that is so important is DRINK WATER! This is absolutely vital for any diet that you're on, and you need it if not on one as well. However, this vital tip is crucial on a keto diet because when you are eating fewer carbs, you are storing less water, meaning that you are going to get dehydrated very easily. You should aim for more than the daily amount of water however, remember that drinking too much water can be fatal as your kidneys can only handle so much as once. While this has mostly happened to soldiers in the military, it does happen to dieters as well, so it is something to be aware of.

Along with that same tip is to keep your electrolytes. You have three major electrolytes in your body. When you are on a keto diet, your body is reducing the amount of water that you store. It can be flushing out the electrolytes that your body needs as well, and this can make you sick. Some of the ways that you can fight this are by either salting your food or drinking bone broth. You can also eat pickled vegetables.

Eat when you're hungry instead of snacking or eating constantly. This is also going to help, and when you focus on natural foods and health foods, this will help you even more. Eating processed foods is the worst thing you can do for fighting cravings, so you should really get into the routine of trying to eat whole foods instead.

Another routine that you can get into is setting a note somewhere that you can see it that will remind you of why you're doing this in the first place and why it's important to you. Dieting is hard, and you will have moments of weakness where you're wondering why you are doing this. Having a reminder will help you feel better, and it can really help with your perspective.

Tracking progress is something that straddles the fence. A Lot of people say that this helps a lot of people and you can celebrate your wins, however, as everyone is different and they have different goals, progress can be slower in some than others. This can cause others to be frustrated and sad, as well as wanting to give up. One of the most important things to remember is that while progress takes time, and you shouldn't get discouraged if you don't see results right away. With most diets, it takes at least a month to see any results. So don't get discouraged and keep trying if your body is saying that you can. If you can't, then you will need to talk to your doctor and see if something else is for you.

You should make it a daily routine to try and lower your stress. Stress will not allow you to get into ketosis, which is that state that keto wants to put you in. The reason for this being that stress increases the hormone known as cortisol in your blood, and it will prevent your body from being able to burn fats for energy. This is because your body has too much sugar in your blood. If you're going through a really high period of stress right now in your life, then this diet is not a great idea. Some great ideas for this would be getting into the habit or routine of taking the time to do something relaxing, such as walking and making sure that you're getting enough sleep, leads to another routine that you need to do.

You need to get enough sleep. This is so important not just for your diet but also for your mind and body as well. Poor sleep also raises those stress hormones that can cause issues for you, so you need to get into the routine of getting seven hours of sleep at night on the minimum and nine hours if you can. If you're getting less than this, you need to change the routine you have in place right now and make sure that you establish a new routine where you are getting more sleep. As a result, your health and diet will be better.

Another routine that you need to get into is to give up diet soda and sugar substitutes. This is going to help you with your diet as well because diet soda can actually increase your sugar levels to a bad amount, and most diet sodas contain aspartame. This can be a carcinogen, so it's actually quite dangerous. Another downside is that using these sugar substitutes just makes you want more sugar . Instead, you need to get into the habit of drinking water or sparkling water if you like the carbonation.

Staying consistent is another routine that you need to get yourself into. No matter what you are choosing to do, make sure it's something that you can actually do. Try a routine for a couple of weeks and make serious notes of mental and physical problems that you're going through as well as any emotional issues that come your way. Make changes as necessary until you find something that works well for you and that you can stick to it. Remember that you need to give yourself time to get used to this and time to get used to changes before you give up on them.

Be honest with yourself, as well. This is another big tip for this diet. If you're not honest with yourself, this isn't going to work. Another reason that you need to be honest with yourself is if something isn't working you need to be able to understand that and change it. Are you giving yourself enough time to make changes? Are you pushing too hard? If so, you need to understand what is going on with yourself and how you need to deal with the changes that you're going through. Remember not to get upset or frustrated. This diet takes time, and you need to be able to be a little more patient to make this work effectively.

Getting into the routine of cooking for yourself is also going to help you so much on this diet. Eating out is fun, but honestly, on this diet, it can be hard to eat out. It is possible to do so with a little bit of special ordering and creativity, but you can avoid all the trouble by simply cooking for yourself. It saves time, and it saves a lot of cash.

This another topic falls into both the tip and routine category. Get into the habit of cleaning your kitchen. It's very hard to stick to a diet if your kitchen is dirty and full of junk food.

Clear out the junk (donate it if you can, even though it's junk, there are tons of hungry people that would appreciate it) and replace all of the bad food with healthy keto food instead. Many people grab the carbs like crazy because they haven't cleared out their cabinets, and it's everywhere they look. Remember, with this diet, no soda, pasta, bread, candy, and things of that nature. Replacing your food with healthy food and making a regular routine of cleaning your kitchen and keeping the bad food out is going to help you be more successful with your diet, which is what you want here.

Getting into the routine of having snacks on hand is a good idea as well. This keeps you from giving into temptation while you're out, and you can avoid reaching for that junk food. You can make sure that they are healthy, and you will be sticking to your high-intensity diet, which is what you want. There are many different keto snacks that you can use for yourself and to eat. We will have a list of recipes in the following phases to help this as well.

A good tip would be to use keto sticks or a glucose meter. This will give you feedback on whether your users do this diet right. The best option here is a glucose meter. It's expensive, but it's the most accurate. Be aware that if you use ketostix, they are cheaper, but the downside is that they are not accurate enough to help you. A perfect example is that they have a habit of telling people their ketone count is low when they are actually the opposite.

Try not to overeat as this will throw you out of where you need to be. Get into the routine of paying attention to what you're eating and how much. If this is something that you're struggling with, try investing in a food scale. You will be able to see exactly what it is your eating and make sure that your understanding your portions and making sure you stay in ketosis.

Another tip is to make sure that you're improving your gut health. This is so important. Your gut is pretty much linked to every other system in your body, so make sure that this something that you want to take seriously. When you have healthy gut flora, your body's hormones, along with your insulin sensitivity and metabolic flexibility will all be more efficient. When your flexibility is functioning at an optimal level, your body is able to adapt to your diet easier. If it's not, then it will convert the fat your trying to use for energy into body fat.

Batch cooking or meal prepping is another routine that is a good thing to get into. This is an especially good routine for on the go women. When you cook in batches, you are able to make sure that you have meals that are ready to go, and you don't have to cook every single day, and you can save a lot of time as well. You will also be making your environment better for your diet because you're supporting your goals instead of working against them.

The last tip is to mention exercise again. Getting into the routine of exercising can boost your ketone levels, and it can help you with your issues on transitioning to keto. Exercises also use different types of energy for your fuel that you need. When your body gets rid of the glycogen storages, it needs other forms of energy, and it will turn into that energy that you need. Just remember to avoid exercises that are going to hurt you. Stay in the smaller exercises and lower intensity.

Following these tips and getting into these routines is going to help you stay on track and make sure that your diet will go as smoothly as it possibly can.

CHAPTER 12. HOW THE KETO DIET AFFECTS 50 YEARS OLD WOMEN

All women know it is much more difficult for women to lose weight than it is for men to lose weight. A woman will live on a starvation level diet and exercise like a triathlete and only lose five pounds. A man will stop putting dressing on his salad and will lose twenty pounds. It just is not fair. But we have the fact that we are women to blame. Women naturally have more standing between them and weight loss than men do.

The mere fact that we are women is the largest single contributor to the reason we find it difficult to lose weight. Since our bodies always think they need to be prepared for the possibility of pregnant women will naturally have more body fat and less mass in our muscles than men will. Muscle cells burn more calories than fat cells do. So because we are women we will always lose weight more slowly than men will.

Being in menopause will also cause women to add more pounds to their bodies, especially in the lower half of the body. After menopause, a woman's metabolism naturally slows down. Your hormone levels will decrease. These two factors alone will cause weight gain in the post-menopausal woman.

Women are a direct product of their hormones. Men also have hormones but not the ones like we have that regulate every function in our bodies. And the hormones in women will fluctuate around their everyday habits like lack of sleep, poor eating habits, and menstrual cycles. These hormones cause women to crave sweets around the time their periods occur. These cravings will wreck any diet plan. Staying true to the keto plan is challenging at this time because of the intense craving for sweets and carbs. Also having your period will often make you feel and look bloated because of the water your body holds onto during this time. And having cramps make you more likely to reach for a bag of cookies than a plate of steak and salad.

Because we are women we may experience challenges on the keto diet that men will not face because they are men. One of these challenges is having weight loss plateau or even experiencing weight gain. This can happen because of the influence of hormones on weight loss in women. If this happens you will want to increase your consumption of good fats like ghee, butter, eggs, coconut oil, beef, avocados, and olive oil. Any food that is cooked or prepared using oil must be prepared in olive oil or avocado oil.

You can also use MCT oil. MCT stands for medium-chain triglycerides. This is a form of fatty acid that is saturated and has many health benefits. MCT can help with many body functions from weight loss to improved brain function. MCTs are mostly missing from the typical American diet because we have been told that saturated fats are harmful to the body, and as a group they are. But certain saturated fats, like MCTs, are actually beneficial to the body, especially when they come from good foods like beef or coconut oil. They are easier to digest than most other saturated fats and may help improve heart and brain function and prevent obesity.

Many women on a keto diet will struggle with imbalances in their hormones. On the keto diet, you do not rely on lowered calories to lose weight but on foods' effect on your hormones. So when women begin the keto diet any issues they are already having with their hormones will be brought to attention and may cause the woman to give up before she really begins. Always remember that the keto diet is responsible for cleansing the system first so that the body can easily respond to the wonderful effects a keto diet has to offer.

Do not try to work toward the lean body that many men sport. It is best for an overall function that women stay at twenty-two to twenty-six percent body fat. Our hormones will function best in this range and we can't possibly function without our hormones. Women who are very lean, like gymnasts and extreme athletes, will find their hormones no longer function or function at a less than optimal rate. And remember that ideal weight may not be the right weight for you. Many women find that they perform their best when they are at their happy weight. If you find yourself fighting with yourself to lose the last few pounds you think you need to lose in order to have the perfect body then it may not be worth it. The struggle will affect your hormone function. Carefully observing the keto diet will allow time for your hormones to stabilize and regulate themselves back to their pre-obesity normal function.

Like any other diet plan, the keto diet will work better if you are active. Regular exercise will allow the body to strengthen and tone muscles and will help to work off excess fat reserves. But exercise requires energy to accomplish. If you restrict your carb intake too much you might not have the energy needed to be physically able to make it all the way through the day and still be able to maintain an exercise routine. You might need to add in more carbs to your diet through the practice of carb cycling.

As a woman, you know that sometimes your emotions get the better of you. This is true with your body, as you well know, and can be a major reason why women find it extremely difficult at times to lose weight the way they want to lose weight. We have been led to believe that not only can we do it all but that we must do it all. This gives many women unnecessary levels of pressure and can cause them to engage in emotional eating. Some women might have lowered feelings of self-worth and may not feel they are entitled to the benefits of the keto diet, and turning to food relieves the feelings of inadequacy that we try to hide from the world.

When you engage in the same activity for a long period of time it becomes a habit. When you reach for the bag of potato chips or the tub of ice cream whenever you are angry, upset, or depressed, then your brain will eventually tell you to reach for food whenever you feel an emotion that you don't want to deal with. Food acts as a security blanket against the world outside. It may be necessary to address any extreme emotional issues you are having before you begin the keto diet so that you are better assured of success.

The basic act of staying on the keto diet can be very challenging for some women. Many women see beginning a new diet to lose weight as a punishment for being overweight. It may be worthwhile for you to work at changing the settings of your mind if you are feeling this way. You may need to remind yourself daily that the keto diet is not a punishment but a blessing for your body. Tell yourself that you are not denying yourself certain foods because you can't eat them, but because you do not like the way those foods make your body feel. Don't watch other people eating their high carb diet and pity yourself. Instead, feel sorry for the people who have trapped themselves in a high-calorie diet and are not experiencing the benefits that you are experiencing.

And for the first thirty days cut out all sweeteners, even the non-sugar ones that are allowed on the keto diet. While they may make food taste better they also remind your brain that it needs sweet foods when it really doesn't. Cutting them out for at least thirty days will break the cycle that your body has fallen into and will cut the cravings for sweets in your diet.

It is very possible for women to be successful on the keto diet if they are prepared to follow a few simple adjustments that will make the diet look differently than your male partner might be eating but that will make you successful in the long run.

During the first one or two weeks, you will need to consume extra fat than a man might need to. Doing this will have three important effects on your body. First, it will cause your mitochondria to intensify their acceptance of your new way of finding energy. Mitochondria are tiny organisms that are found in cells and are responsible for using the fuel that insulin brings to the cell for fuel for the cell. Increasing your fat intake will also help make sure you are getting enough calories in your daily diet. This is important because if your body thinks you are starving it will begin to conserve calories and you will stop losing weight.

The third benefit from eating more fat, and perhaps the most important, is the psychological boost you will get from seeing that you can eat more fat and still lose weight and feel good. It will also reset your mindset that you previously might have held against fat. For so long we have been told that low fat is the only way to lose weight. But an absence of dietary fat will lead to overeating and binge eating out of a feeling of deprivation. When you begin the diet by allowing yourself to eat a lot, or too much in your mind, fat, then you swing the pendulum around to the other side of the fat scale where it properly belongs. You teach yourself that fat can be good for you. Increasing the extra intake of fats should not last beyond the second week of the diet. Your body will improve its ability to create and burn ketones and body fat, and then you will begin using your own body fat for fuel and you can begin to lower your reliance on dietary fat a little bit so that you will begin to lose weight.

The keto diet is naturally lower in calories if you follow the recommended levels of food intake. It is not necessary to try to restrict your intake of calories even further. All you need to do is to eat only until you are full and not one bite more. Besides losing weight the aim of the keto diet is to retrain your body on how to work properly. You will need to learn to trust your body and the signals it sends out to be able to readjust to a proper way of eating. So don't feel you need to consume every bite on your plate. If having leftovers bothers you then make just one portion for each person to consume and no more. Left to its own devices your body systems will properly regulate themselves and this includes the intake of food. Give the keto diet a chance to work properly.

CONCLUSION

Thank you for making it through to the end of *Keto After 50: The Ultimate Guide to Ketogenic Diet for Men and Women Over 50,* let's hope it was informative and able to provide you with all of the tools you need to achieve your goals whatever they may be.

Beginning the Keto diet can seem daunting at first, but you have all of the information you need to help you get started! I hope that you find the courage and motivation to follow your new lifestyle so that you can experience all of the incredible benefits that come with the diet.

If you ever have any questions, feel free to use this book as your ultimate guide. There are going to be bumps along the way, but you are very well prepared at this point. Remember that there is no point in giving up! The Ketogenic Diet works, the science is proof! As long as you follow the rules, keep your carbs to a minimum, and eat the foods you are supposed to, you are going to see the results in no time! All you have to do is put in the work!

Finally, if you found this book useful in any way, a review on Amazon is always appreciated!

CPSIA information can be obtained
at www.ICGtesting.com
Printed in the USA
LVHW080507100121
676040LV00001B/19